Multiple Sclerosis

This book explains exactly what M.S. is and describes the things you can do which may stop you getting worse. It includes advice on nutrition for the central nervous system, exercise, yoga, posture, incontinence, fatigue, relationships and sex, and perhaps most important of all, full details about the evening primrose oil, a dietary supplement shown to be effective for many people with M.S.

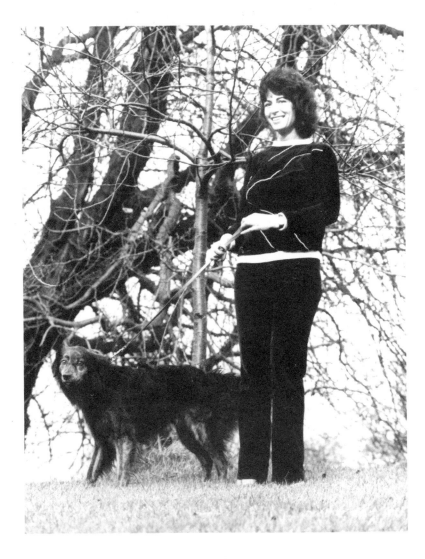

Judy Graham
Photo: John Kelly

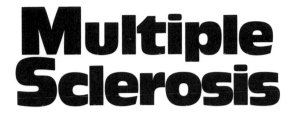

Multiple Sclerosis

A Self-help Guide to Its Management

by

JUDY GRAHAM

THORSONS PUBLISHERS LIMITED
Wellingborough, Northamptonshire

First published 1981

British Library Cataloguing in Publication Data

Graham, Judy
  Multiple sclerosis.
  1. Multiple sclerosis.
  2. Self-care, Health
  I. Title
  616.8'34068   RC377

  ISBN 0-7225-0625-2
  ISBN 0-7225-0624-4 Pbk

Filmset by Specialised Offset Services Ltd., Liverpool
Printed in Great Britain by Whitstable Litho Ltd., Whitstable, Kent

CONTENTS

ACKNOWLEDGEMENTS

This book could not have been written without the help of a great many people. Very little in it is original material: I have simply gathered into one place all the various bits and pieces about the management of M.S. which have been written by other people elsewhere.

The greatest help has come from ARMS and its chairman John Simkins. It is only through being a member of ARMS that all the information has come my way. I have also taken freely from some of the ARMS Education Service booklets.

Particular thanks are due to Joe Osborne, of the Burton and South Derbyshire Independent Pool, for giving me the inspiration to do a follow-up to his own book, and for information in Chapter 14 on exercise.

Many doctors have helped me with research material, books, and verbal advice. Some have written books of their own which are listed at the end. My thanks to: Dr Helmut J. Bauer; Dr Elizabeth Forsythe; Dr Michael Crawford; Professor Roy Swank; Professor E.J. Field; Dr Paul Evers; Dr Ahmed Hassam; Drs Alexander and Penelope Burnfield; Dr David F. Horrobin; Dr Jurgen Mertin; Dr Paula Dore-Duffy; Professor W. Ritchie-Russell; Dr Len Mervyn; Dr John Mansfield.

For their help with particular chapters, my thanks to: Sally O'Connor; Judith Harding; John Williams; Leslie Smith; Howard Kent; John Sullivan; Gill Robinson; Uta Greiner; Ahmed Hussein; Morag MacDougall; Rita Greer; Roger MacDougall; M.S. Society of Canada; Gilbert MacDonald and the M.S. Society of Great Britain and Northern Ireland.

I would also like to thank Vivien Neves for reading the manuscript and for writing the Foreword to this book, and her husband John Kelly for taking the photograph of me which appears on the frontispiece.

FOREWORD

I was diagnosed with M.S. earlier this year at the age of 32, after four years of worry and not knowing what was wrong with me. At first I felt relieved that they'd given my wretched illness a name. But then I wondered what to do about it.

Judy Graham gave me the manuscript of her book to read after the news of my illness appeared in the newspapers. It told me everything I wanted to know or ask about M.S. which I didn't understand from my doctor. It's easy to read, and takes the mystery out of the illness.

The most important chapters to me have been the ones on diet, essential fatty acids, evening primrose oil, and relaxation. Personally, I now follow the Swank low-fat diet, which I feel has stabilized my own condition. I've also started taking evening primrose oil capsules.

And it was with relief and pleasure that I read the frank chapter on the usually taboo subject of relationships and sex which are, after all, very important to us all.

As it's so often harder for the family of an M.S. sufferer to accept and cope with the illness, I think this book should be read not only by those with M.S., but by their families too. It should take away some of the fear surrounding M.S., and enable people like myself to lead a happier life.

VIVIEN NEVES
December 1980

Vivien Neves is a top model, and is the only one ever to appear nude in The Times. *She was diagnosed as suffering from Multiple Sclerosis in 1980. She is married with a daughter.*

PREFACE

The origins of this book began back in 1974. That was the year when I was diagnosed as having M.S., at the age of twenty-seven, though my first symptoms started when I was about twenty-four. It was also the year when the Multiple Sclerosis Action Group began. I, with about a dozen or so other people, were its founder members and we held our inaugural meeting in my London flat.

Those people all had one thing in common. We either had M.S. ourselves, or were married to someone with it. Just as important, we were a group of very angry activists who were outraged and enraged that nothing could be done for us. So we decided to do something for ourselves.

This book, in a way, is the fruit of the work of this self-help action group over the last six years. I certainly could not have written it unless I had been an active member of that group (now called ARMS – Action for Research into Multiple Sclerosis).

Much of that work was to do with research. By a series of, to my way of thinking, lucky and inspired choices, ARMS became associated with Professor E.J. Field in Newcastle. We raised money to fund a unit for him, where he has been doing some valuable research into essential fatty acids and M.S. Not long after, ARMS also became associated with Dr Michael Crawford at the Nuffield Laboratories of Comparative Medicine in Regents Park, London. His research, though quite separate from Professor Field's, seemed to dovetail nicely with it. His main research was about brain lipids, and when we arrived on the scene, he extended his research to investigate a diet for people with M.S. which was rich in essential fatty acids.

I was lucky – and forthright – enough to be a guinea pig for both doctors. My arm was proffered many a time for blood tests. I believe my initials, plus some tables I do not fully comprehend, are published in some medical papers reporting their work.

Professor Field was testing what was happening to my blood as a result of taking *Naudicelle* capsules of evening primrose oil. Dr Crawford was testing my blood to see what difference a diet high in essential fatty acids would make (I was on evening primrose oil capsules at the same time).

My visits to Dr Crawford were always a delight. His laboratories overlook London Zoo and are right next to the parrot house. So it was not like an appointment with any other doctor. No one there wore white coats, I was on first-name terms with everyone, and at no time was I treated like a 'patient'. I was what is known as a 'highly-motivated participant'. I was told to eat a diet of foods like liver, fish, lean meat, spinach, fresh fruit and vegetables. Apart from the occasional gross misdemeanour, like chocolate mousse or cream cake, I stuck pretty closely to his diet, and still do.

The result of those two tests was that my blood changed from abnormal to normal in its composition of essential fatty acids. By Professor Field's diagnostic test, it no longer gives an M.S. reading.

However, there is no doubt that I still have M.S. Yet, I am better now than I was six years ago. Then, I felt like I was wearing wellington boots up to my thighs while walking through a quagmire in the Arctic Circle. Now, I can wear high-heel shoes without toppling over, and the ground feels like real ground under my feet, although I do still occasionally get 'prickly' hands and feet, dodgy eyesight, cold legs and feet, and fatigue. I can still walk the dog briskly across Hampstead Heath, but I would be pushing my luck to sprint across a road.

I can't claim any of the spectacular improvements of people like Roger MacDougall or Alan Greer who have been photo-graphed balancing on one leg, waving from ladders, or cavorting along heathland or beaches. Mine is not a dramatic story. Quite honestly, anyone who has known me over the years would not notice any difference. Many people I meet do not even know I have M.S.

Doctors could easily say that my improvement must mean I

am in a remission, but this is not so. I have never had the relapsing/remitting pattern of the disease. I have the type where there is some symptom or other present all the time. M.S. is known to be a degenerative disease, yet I have got no worse; in fact, I have got better. So I, at least, am convinced I must be doing something right, something to stabilize my condition.

That something is very likely to be a combination of the evening primrose oil and the low-fat diet rich in essential fatty acids, both of which I have followed now for years; but exercise and yoga have been valuable too.

The idea of exercise as a therapy for M.S. comes from Joe Osborne. Joe runs the Burton and South Derbyshire Independent Pool for the Sufferers of Multiple Sclerosis. He has been organizing weekly gym classes for people with M.S. for a few years, with impressive results. All the members were also taking *Naudicelle* capsules of evening primrose oil, and a diet high in essential fatty acids and low in animal fat. Joe himself wrote the forerunner to this book, which is full of heartening testimonials about the success of this combined therapy.

Since learning of their success, I have joined a swish London gym kitted out with sophisticated equipment to tone up flabby tummies, dropped bottoms and superfluous sag. That is what most women go there for, but I can testify that it works too for building up stamina and muscle strength and increasing fitness.

I also practise yoga and cannot praise it too highly. A few years ago the Yoga for Health Foundation got in touch with ARMS, and since then they have been running special classes for people with M.S., with some excellent improvements. I joined the Foundation, and now go to one of their ordinary classes in London. I usually turn up at the class tired, but by the end of it I am full of energy and feel a general sense of well-being.

For the record, I have also had a go at some of the other things in this book too. For more than one will-powered year I stuck to a gluten-free diet until profiteroles at a wedding put an end to it. I have never felt healthier than when I was on that diet, and if I could muster the will-power I would go back on it.

I have also done the whole boring food allergy test. I

discovered, by an arduous process of trial and error, that I was allergic to yeast, cane sugar, milk, egg yolks, peanuts and coffee; but my attempts to exclude these foods have been singularly unsuccessful. The truth is, I would rather eat them and suffer the consequences than give them up, although I would recommend to others a sterner approach if you want to feel completely well again.

I should also add that I have been treated by an acupuncturist ever since I was diagnosed, and have recently started having deep-massage treatment once a fortnight. Both have helped.

With this all-embracing approach, people often ask me, in exasperated tones, how I know which one is doing me any good. This would be a reasonable question if I was conducting some scientific experiment on myself, but I am not. I'm simply trying to do the things that just might stabilize my condition, and in that I've been eminently successful.

'Clutching at straws' is the other old favourite I'm assailed with. Yet this is a quite inappropriate analogy as straws are supposed to be for drowning people, and I'm quite safely on dry land.

In this book, I am passing on details of the things which I have found to be of help to me, plus some other information which I have not needed for myself but others may find useful.

That is really why I have written this book. I felt it was uniquely up to me to write it. I know of no one else who has M.S., who has been privileged enough to test all the therapies, who has direct access to all the research scientists, who is well enough to tell the tale, and who has the professional skills to execute it. Having gained a degree in Modern History, and then working as a newspaper journalist and television researcher, I am used to researching, collecting and sifting vast amounts of information, and putting complex issues into clear and simple language. I make no apologies for this being written in layman's language, as that is who it is for.

If I had written this book six years ago, there would no doubt have been a venomous chapter somewhere about doctors, neurologists in particular, who in my experience were remote, arrogant, and totally lacking in helpful advice of any sort. My one and only stay in a neurological ward provided ample proof of this. In order to make a diagnosis, the National

Hospital used what seemed the entire armoury of their technological equipment. Despite all that, I felt as though I might as well have been living in the Dark Ages, for all the help modern medicine could offer me.

The time I spent in a ward, of what is considered to be the top-notch neurological hospital in Britain, was nothing short of dire. I have never felt so ill in all my life as the week following the lumbar puncture. In fact, the whole episode in hospital was so thoroughly unpleasant that I resolved never to be a hospital patient again.

Those were the feelings of six years ago, though I have not bothered to see a neurologist since as a patient as there seemed no point. In general, however, my attitude towards doctors has mellowed over the years. Since then, I genuinely believe that doctors and scientists have stepped up their efforts into finding a prevention, cause, treatment and cure for M.S. I would like to think that ARMS has had some effect on gingering up the medicos, and everyone else.

Through ARMS open meetings and research seminars, I have been lucky enough to meet some of the scientists involved in M.S. research, even including some very pleasant neurologists. It has been a heartening experience. I have found them to be concerned and compassionate people genuinely motivated to solve the problem of M.S., and who have valued the pressure (and funds) a self-help group like ARMS can bring to bear on a particular field of research.

My own G.P., a young woman of about the same age as me, has been encouraging and supportive of everything I have been doing. I think I am her only patient with M.S. and every so often I present her with a wodge of research data which she accepts and reads enthusiastically.

Even though I am a lay person, it is highly likely that my experience of M.S. exceeds that of most General Practitioners. Through my membership of ARMS and the M.S. Society, I have met hundreds of people with M.S. in every possible stage of the disease. I have also been involved in the production of two BBC television documentaries about M.S.

My involvement with the disease is not such a full-time pre-occupation as it might sound. Since I was diagnosed, I have travelled round the U.S.A. with a television film crew, been a radio reporter, a radio producer, a Fleet Street feature writer, a BBC television producer, and travelled all round Australia (via Bangkok and Singapore), plus a host of other countries, on my own with a tape recorder. While writing this book I have been doing fairly gruelling work as a radio producer and reporter.

It would be misleading, though, to give the impression that M.S. has not affected my life in a damaging way. There is no doubt that it has. Insecurity has become a fact of life. At the moment my way of earning a living involves all the things which are most precariously at risk with M.S.: legwork; manual dexterity; 100 per cent concentration; brain power; long, hard hours; the ability to work fast under pressure; and a good, articulate microphone voice.

By revealing that I have M.S. I have been debarred from being taken onto the pensionable staff of the television company I used to work for, and so I am forced to fall back entirely on my own wits and resources and make a living as a freelance.

Since I cannot afford to give up my livelihood, I cannot afford to get worse. Certainly one of my motives in pursuing all these therapies is to keep the social handicaps as well as the physical ones to a minimum.

It has taken the best part of six years to collect all this knowledge together. I certainly wish that a book such as this had existed when I knew nothing of M.S. back in 1974. My hope is that this book will satisfy a sorely-felt need, particularly from newly-diagnosed people all over the world. If doctors are failing to fulfil this need, then we must do it ourselves.

JUDY GRAHAM

Note: I should make it clear that I do not have any financial, business interest or other reward in any of the companies listed in this book.

INTRODUCTION

This book is for people who have been diagnosed as having M.S., and for their families, friends and helpers.

When first diagnosed as having M.S., few people have any idea what it is, or what can be done to help it. Your doctor is likely to tell you, 'Go away and forget about it' or 'I'm sorry, there's nothing we can do for you'. If he tells you, 'Come back if anything happens and we'll help you', it is equally misleading.

To be fair, there is quite a lot your doctor can do to help you. You know by now that there is no cure for M.S., and no treatment; but there are still some things he can do for you which will have a good effect on certain symptoms. He can prescribe ACTH if you get an attack, or certain drugs to help with things like bladder urgency or retention, or spasms. It is certainly worth going to see your doctor when a new symptom crops up and getting as much help from him as possible.

But anything your doctor gives you can only be a palliative. Unless he is very forward-thinking, he is unlikely to tell you the kind of things you need to know to *manage* the disease. Things about diet, exercise, rest and mental outlook.

This is what this book is about – the *management* of Multiple Sclerosis.

I cannot claim this 'regime' has been put to any strict scientific test. But there are many hundreds of M.S. people who, in a haphazard sort of way, have been doing all or at least some of the things suggested in this book and have felt much better for it.

This management of M.S. has two great virtues. Firstly, it is about self-help. That means *you* decide to do something to help yourself, rather than have others do things for you. That decision to help yourself will make you feel much more positive.

Secondly, the management 'regime' is a very healthy way of life and can only do you good. Do not worry that it has not been subjected to rigorous double-blind trials. Those trials – apart from testing to see whether something works – are also to test the toxicity and effectiveness of drugs. Since the management of Multiple Sclerosis does not involve the use of drugs, there are none of those risks.

However, do take your doctor into your confidence. If you are going to start a special diet, or go on polyunsaturated fatty acid capsules, or take up gym or yoga, please tell your doctor what you are doing, if only to let him know why you are bounding into his surgery next time you do!

1   THE MANAGEMENT OF MULTIPLE SCLEROSIS

Here you are, landed with a disease with no known cause, no known cure, and no known treatment.

You could languish in a private hell and lament your terrible lot, or you could decide to do everything in your power to fight the disease and help yourself.

Methods of Approach
The full armoury of weapons with which to wage war on M.S. includes all of the following:

—— Supplementing your diet with essential fatty acids (evening primrose oil) plus vitamins and minerals.
—— Eating a healthy, low-fat diet, rich in essential fatty acids.
—— Doing daily exercise or physiotherapy.
—— Maintaining a positive attitude to life.
—— Keeping your brain active and stimulated.
—— Getting enough rest.
—— Avoiding fatigue.
—— Leading a stress-free life.
—— Having satisfying relationships with other people.

If you could do all of those, you would surely be a happy person, and as healthy as possible. But unless you are superhuman, it is probably asking a bit much to keep up all of them all of the time.

However, if you can manage just the first three, with as much of the others as possible when possible, you would be doing a lot to keep yourself as fit and healthy as possible.

Make an Early Start

The earlier you can start, the better. Studies have shown that the people who benefit most from this self-help regime are the recently-diagnosed. The progress of the disease seems to be delayed, or even arrested. I know that claims like this are notoriously hard to prove in a disease like M.S., where symptoms come and go and nobody can tell you exactly why, but even without cast iron proof, there are enough personal testimonies from enough people for you to know that this regime has been associated with some very encouraging results. Even more seriously disabled people have noticed an all-round improvement in health, and an arresting, or reversal, of some symptoms. Do not wait until you get worse before you decide to try this self-help programme, and if you decide to wait until it all has the green light from the medical men, you could be waiting a very long time.

I must stress that *nothing in this book is suggested as being a cure.*

There is still no cure for M.S. Nor is anything suggested as a treatment. To be a treatment, it would need to have undergone more rigorous scientific trials than anything in this book has done.

The best one can hope for at the moment is a *management* of the disease. That means doing the things that are good for you, that might make you feel better instead of worse, and that give you a chance of enjoying life to the full.

2 WHAT EXACTLY IS M.S.?

If you know what is going on in this disease, it is easier to understand why the self-help management programme is relevant.

Multiple Sclerosis is a disease which affects the brain and the spinal cord, which are together known as the central nervous system (C.N.S.). The damage to the C.N.S. occurs in many widely scattered areas. That is why it is called 'multiple' – there are many patches of damage. The damaged area is filled with hard material, or scars. 'Sclerosis' means scars.

The Central Nervous System

The C.N.S. has two main types of tissue in it: grey matter and white matter. The *grey matter* is called that because it looks grey to the naked eye. This is the part of the brain where thinking, computing, organizing, and memory takes place. M.S. has little or no effect on the grey matter although it does interfere with communication between different parts of the grey matter, with intellectual deterioration at later stages of the disease.

The *white matter* looks white to the naked eye. It consists of fibres which carry messages from the sense organs – like the skin, eyes, ears – up to the higher parts of the brain. The white matter also carries messages from the brain down to the muscles. The white matter also links up various parts of the brain. It is the sort of 'wiring' of the brain, and it is this part that is affected by the patches of scarring – or Multiple Sclerosis. That is why your ability to feel, move and co-ordinate is affected.

If you feel pins and needles in your hands, or you are dragging your left foot, remember that the trouble is not in either your hand or foot, but in your central nervous system.

How is the Central Nervous System Damaged?

The white areas of the C.N.S. are very similar to an electrical cable containing many wires. Each wire consists of a central core (nerve fibre) which carries electrical impulses. In a cable, it is very important that the wires should not make contact with each other. To stop this happening, each wire is covered by some insulating material – usually rubber or plastic. The insulation makes sure the electricity in the wire goes to its destination without short-circuiting sideways.

Myelin

In the white matter of the C.N.S. each nerve fibre is surrounded by a layer of insulation made mainly of a fatty material known as *myelin*. Without the myelin, nerve signals cannot travel normally, and there may be faulty connections between adjacent nerve fibres.

In M.S. the first process seems to be the destruction of this myelin coating around the nerve fibres. This interferes with the way in which the fibres work. The body then makes the damage worse by attempting to repair the damage, much as it would a skin wound. The damaged area is filled with hard material known as connective tissue (scars or scleroses), which cannot conduct nerve impulses.

Relapses and Remissions

The disease usually consists of a series of attacks, and periods of remission. Each attack usually leaves the M.S. patient a little worse than before. No one knows why the damage stops. During a remission, something – if only we knew exactly what – has switched off the disease process.

When an exacerbation occurs, it means that the myelin in

the white matter in part of the C.N.S. is being destroyed. Nearby areas, although not actually damaged themselves, are affected. For a temporary period, they may fail to function, while the body's repair process is going on.

So, at the height of a relapse, three types of damage to the working of the C.N.S. are going on:

1. Total destruction of the myelin in some fibres which will never recover.
2. Partial destruction of the myelin in some fibres which may be capable of successful repair.
3. Temporary loss of function in nearby fibres whose myelin is basically intact.

Once the attack is over, only the first damage is left, and this may be very small.

'By-Pass' Routes

It may be that when part of the brain is damaged, the function carried out by that part is taken over by other parts of the brain, rather like taking the A1 when the M1 is closed to traffic. It may be that this is happening spontaneously during a remission. You can also be trained to develop by-pass routes in physiotherapy.

3   ESSENTIAL FATTY ACIDS

Many different sorts of fat are essential to the body, but the body can make most of these itself. However, one small group, known as the essential fatty acids, cannot, for the most part, be made in the body, so they must be taken in the food you eat.

In a way, 'fat' is a misleading term for this nutrient. Essential fatty acids (E.F.A.s) are more like proteins, or vitamins, because it is vital you eat them in your food to remain healthy.

E.F.A.s are present in every cell of your body. Roughly 60 per cent of the structure of the brain is this kind of fat, and E.F.A.s are vital for the proper growth and development of the brain and the central nervous system.

For everyone, fats are an essential part of nutrition. They give energy; help to maintain body temperature; insulate the nerves; cushion and protect the tissues; are part of the cell structure of every cell in your body, and are vital for metabolism.

Essential Fatty Acids and Multiple Sclerosis
E.F.A.s are particularly essential for people with M.S. They are needed for the growth and repair of the nervous tissue, and

for the maintenance of its structure. This is particularly important in M.S., where the central nervous system is under attack. If the body lacks these nutrients, any repair of damaged tissue is impossible.

Research has shown that the white matter in the brains of people with M.S. is low in E.F.A.s. They are particularly deficient in linoleic acid. There is also a suggestion that people with M.S. have an inability, perhaps inborn, to handle E.F.A.s correctly. Other studies on people with M.S. have shown that the red and white blood cells, the platelets, and the cells of the myelin sheath, are also deficient in E.F.A.s.

E.F.A.s play a fundamental role in all cell membranes of the body. The fluidity and flexibility of the cell membranes depends on how much E.F.A.s the cells have. The activity of lymphocytes (white blood cells) may be dependent on the state of the cell membrane, and will behave differently according to whether a cell membrane is fluid (plenty of E.F.A.s) or rigid (not enough E.F.A.s).

Saturated, Unsaturated, and Polyunsaturated Fats

You have probably seen the word 'polyunsaturated' on cartons of soft margarine, and wondered what it meant. Whether a fat is saturated, unsaturated or polyunsaturated has to do with its biochemical composition, which is fairly complicated. All you really need to know is that poly-unsaturated fats are much better for people with M.S. than any other kind.

Fat is made from smaller components called fatty acids. Fatty acids are chain-like substances, some with short chains, some with long. The chains are of carbon atoms with hydrogen and oxygen atoms attached. The degree of saturation depends on the extent to which they can absorb more hydrogen. Unsaturated fats are capable of picking up other molecules available to them in the system. Saturated fats cannot take any more hydrogen.

Occasionally, the chains may be linked by a double link, or double bond, instead of the more usual single link or single bond. So:

—— If a fatty acid has *no* double bonds it is *saturated*.
—— If a fatty acid has *one* double bond it is *unsaturated*.
—— If it has *two or more* double bonds it is *polyunsaturated*.

Below is an example of a polyunsaturated fatty acid, linoleic acid.

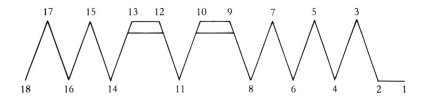

Figure 1. Linoleic acid. This is a chain with 18 carbon atoms and two double bonds.

Saturated Fats
As a rule of thumb, saturated fats tend to be:

—— Hard, solid at room temperature (like butter).
—— Animal fats (e.g. in meat and dairy produce).
—— Need not be taken in the food as the body can make plenty by itself.

Unsaturated and Polyunsaturated Fats
These are usually:

—— Liquid or soft (e.g. vegetable, seed and fish oils).
—— Mostly from fish; vegetables; seeds; offal.
—— Essential to be taken in the diet as the body cannot make enough by itself.

A brief list of the foods rich in unsaturated and poly-unsaturated fats (the same thing as essential fatty acids) includes: sunflower seed oil; safflower seed oil; liver; kidneys; heart; brain; sweetbreads; game; lean meat; dark green leafy vegetables; germinal vegetables; shellfish; fish.

Note: The vegetable oils palm oil and coconut oil are both saturated. Also, unsaturated vegetable or seed oils lose their unsaturated quality when heated, and become like saturated fats. During cooking, the oil is exposed to the oxygen in the air and becomes oxidized, losing its good biological effects.

The higher the temperature, the faster the oxidation. As a guideline, once oil begins to smoke it is too hot and will have become saturated. Moderately hot oil of below smoking temperatures is safe to cook food in. Choose cold-pressed oils as the natural anti-oxidants have not been removed.

Oil should not be re-used in cooking, as it becomes more oxidized and saturated each time it is heated. Vegetable and seed oils are most beneficial eaten uncooked, as salad dressing.

The Families of Essential Fatty Acids

There are two families of essential fatty acids. Both families are very important to the dietary management of M.S. The first family is *linoleic acid* and its derivatives. Strictly speaking, biochemists call this the Omega 6 family and linoleic acid is the head of the family. The second family is *alpha-linolenic acid* and its derivatives. Biochemists call this the Omega 3 family, and alpha-linolenic acid is the parent.

When foods containing these fatty acids are eaten, the body makes longer-chain fatty acids with more double bonds. These longer-chain, more unsaturated fatty acids are more biologically active than the original linoleic acid and alpha-linolenic acid, and it is only these longer-chain fatty acids which are used by the brain.

Foods Rich in the Linoleic Acid Family
Sunflower seed oil; safflower seed oil; evening primrose oil; liver; kidneys; brains; sweetbreads; lean meat; legumes.

Foods Rich in the Alpha-Linolenic Family
Green vegetables; fish; seafood; fish liver oils; linseeds; certain legumes.

The Conversion Process

By means of a complicated biochemical process, the two essential fatty acid families convert into their derivatives. Linoleic acid converts to *arachidonic acid*. Alpha-linolenic acid converts to *cervonic acid*.

Step by step, and vastly oversimplified, the conversion of linoleic acid through to arachidonic acid is shown below.

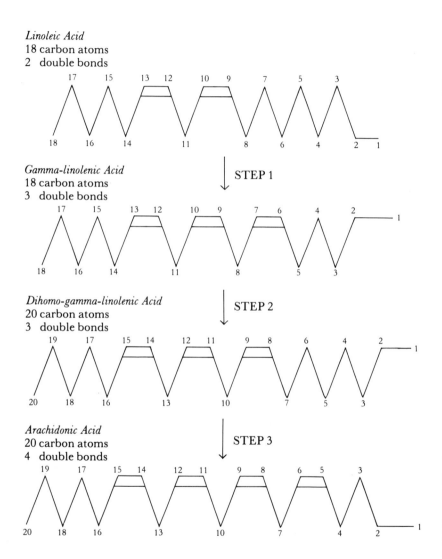

Figure 2. The main stages in the conversion of linoleic acid to arachidonic acid.

Beyond Step 3
Arachidonic acid can then be converted to even more complicated longer chains of unsaturated fatty acids which are essential to the structure of the nervous system.

Arachidonic Acid
Is one of the most important and effective of the essential fatty acids. It plays a vital role in the structure of healthy cells, and is involved in the production of hormones. It may also play a part in the body's immune system.

Arachidonic acid is available in some foods in small quantities (e.g. liver), but most of it has to be manufactured in the body.

If the body is having problems with this manufacturing process, as may be the case in M.S., some way has to be found to get round this problem.

Helping the Conversion Process

In M.S. something somewhere along the line is not working as it should, so that the end-products of the essential fatty acids are not getting through to the places where they are needed.

Even in bodies which are working properly, a lot of the linoleic acid never gets converted to arachidonic acid. It gets used up as energy along the way.

In M.S. it seems that even less is getting through, and the problem seems to lie in Step 1 – linoleic acid to gamma-linolenic acid.

If the problem lies in the conversion of linoleic acid to gamma-linolenic acid, the clever thing would be to jump the first step completely, and start at the second step, gamma-linolenic acid. There seems to be no difficulty in converting from gamma-linolenic acid onwards.

However, research has shown that Step 1 becomes easier if you eat a diet rich in *zinc* (found particularly in seafoods). Indeed, zinc seems to be essential for Step 1. (See Chapter 9 on vitamins and minerals.)

Gamma-Linolenic Acid

This essential fatty acid is 50 per cent more unsaturated than linoleic acid. However, it is not present in any of the commercially-produced vegetable oils. In fact, it is quite rare.

First stages of growth

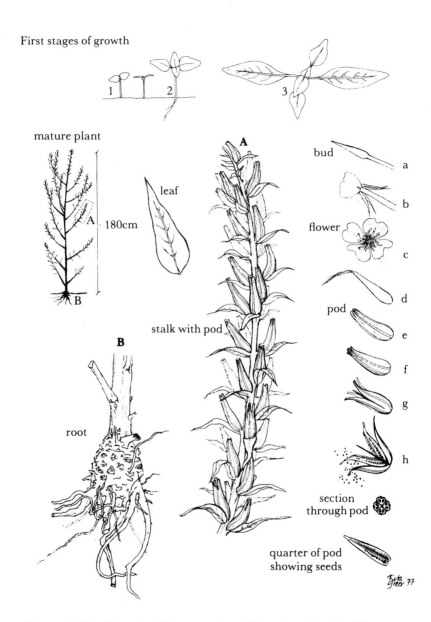

mature plant

180cm

leaf

stalk with pod

root

A

B

bud — a

flower — b

c

pod — d

e

f

g

h

section through pod

quarter of pod showing seeds

Figure 3. The Evening Primrose plant (*Oenothera biennis*). 1-3, young plants with 2, 4 and 6 leaves: a-h, stages in development of flower, pod and seeds. *By kind permission of Rita Greer*.

However, it is found in a prolific plant called the *evening primrose*. Taking the oil from this plant is the best way to make sure the later stages of the biochemical conversion process in the body work properly. (See Chapter 4 on evening primrose oil.)

The Evening Primrose Plant

This plant grows to between five and six feet in height. It has primrose-like petals, which only open in the evenings, so that the yellow flower can be pollinated by moths. Until recently, the plant's tiny seeds were eaten only by birds. In 1949 the seeds were analysed, and the clear pale yellow oil which came out of the seeds was found to contain a high percentage of linoleic acid plus the unique gamma-linolenic acid.

Since the marketing of the evening primrose oil, the plant is now grown in Europe, North and South America, Israel, Hungary, California as well as in the U.K. Experimental growings have also been made in southern Spain, South Australia, New South Wales and elsewhere.

Research has shown that the gamma-linolenic acid in evening primrose oil is efficient in the biochemical conversion process in the body from Step 2 onwards (see Figure 2). It is what happens beyond Step 2 that is so important for people with M.S.

The Later Stages of the Conversion Process

The essential fatty acids have two quite distinct roles in the body. They form part of the structure, the actual building blocks from which cells are made, but they also give rise to very short-lived substances called *prostaglandins* which help to control the way in which the structures work (see Figure 4).

Prostaglandins

Prostaglandins may hold a vital key in the M.S. mystery. They are manufactured from dihomo-gamma-linolenic acid and from arachidonic acid, both of which are made from gamma-linolenic acid, which is found in evening primrose oil.

Prostaglandins are a newly-discovered class of substance. They have a hormone-like character. Like hormones, they act as regulatory substances, and messengers. Unlike hormones, which are normally produced at one gland, prostaglandins are not produced by glands. They are produced and used very locally, as and when they are needed. They are metabolized on site, and used very quickly.

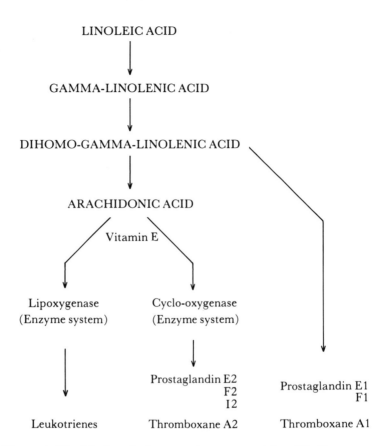

Figure 4. The biochemical conversion process (simplified).

Prostaglandins and Multiple Sclerosis

Prostaglandins have two particularly important functions to do with M.S.: platelet aggregation and regulation of the immune system.

Platelet Aggregation
The platelets are very small particles in the blood. They play a role in blood clotting. In M.S. there is evidence to show that there is an abnormal 'clumping together' of platelets. Prostaglandins are thought to regulate the platelet functions in the blood.

It has been suggested that after several months' treatment of M.S. people with essential fatty acids (taken as evening primrose oil capsules) the platelets in the blood returned to normal. It is thought that prostaglandins, which are metabolized from the E.F.A.s in the capsules, play a vital role in this.

Regulation of the Immune System
There is almost certainly something wrong with the immune system in M.S. The main function of the immune system is to get rid of invading bodies, such as bacteria and viruses, from the body. When the immune system goes wrong, for some reason the body cannot tell the difference between itself, and alien things. In the confusion, the body attacks its own substances.

One line of research at present is based on the hypothesis that the prostaglandins which regulate the immune system may be in short supply in people with M.S. A shortage of prostaglandins (Series 1) leads to defective lymphocytes, and increases the body's susceptibility both to infections and to auto-immune damage (i.e. the body producing antibodies which act against its own tissues).

Prostaglandins (Series 1) may be of critical importance in regulating the function of something called 'T' lymphocytes (white blood cells) and 'T' suppressor cells. 'T' suppressor cells prevent the body from attacking itself. Research has shown that levels of 'T' suppressor cells are very low in M.S. patients during a relapse.

It is known that prostaglandins have the effect of dampening down lymphocytes which are capable of attacking the central nervous system.

Recent Research on Essential Fatty Acids and M.S.
In the last few years, there have been a variety of scientific trials to test the effects of essential fatty acids on patients with M.S.

In 1973, a double-blind trial (Millar and others) showed that sunflower seed oil given to M.S. patients had the effect of reducing both the number and severity of relapses, and of significantly changing the fatty acid composition of the blood.

Later in the 1970s, Professor E.J. Field in Newcastle did some tests to find out the effect of linoleic acid on the lymphocytes of M.S. patients. The lymphocytes are the white blood cells of the lymphatic system. In M.S., there is evidence to show that they are actually attacking the brain. This is part of the auto-immune reaction in M.S. In Professor Field's tests, it was found that linoleic acid had the effect of dramatically inhibiting the lymphocytes in M.S. patients. It was 'dampening down' the lymphocytes, and stopping them attacking the myelin sheath.

In later tests, gamma-linolenic acid was substituted for linoleic acid. The results proved that this more unsaturated fatty acid was superior to linoleic acid: it more rapidly prevented the brain from being attacked. (*Naudicelle* capsules of evening primrose oil were used.)

At about the same time, there was research going on with gamma-linolenic acid at the Nuffield Laboratories in London, by Dr Michael Crawford and Dr Ahmed Hassam. Gamma-linolenic acid was given to M.S. patients (in the form of evening primrose oil capsules) to see what effect it would have on their red blood cells. In M.S. these cells are not only deficient in the essential fatty acids, they are also abnormally large in size and have a poor ability to regulate the passage of fluids through cell membranes. After about eight to ten months of taking gamma-linolenic acid, the red blood cells became normal in all respects.

The conclusion from these and other researchers is that gamma-linolenic acid is capable of altering all abnormal cell membranes, including myelin, and can return them to normal condition in under a year. There is evidence that a dietary supplement of gamma-linolenic acid, taken as evening primrose oil capsules, normalizes the essential fatty acid composition in M.S. patients, and may also stabilize their condition.

4 EVENING PRIMROSE OIL

Evening primrose oil capsules are such an important part of the management programme for M.S. that they deserve a chapter to themselves.

Gamma-Linolenic Acid

Gamma-linolenic acid is the vital 'Step 2' in the biochemical conversion process (Figure 3). It is particularly important that people with M.S. take this, because they are more inefficient than most people at converting from linoleic acid to gamma-linolenic acid in the body. Gamma-linolenic acid is much more powerful than linoleic acid in the conversion process through to arachidonic acid, so it is much more effective than taking sunflower seed oil or safflower seed oil, which contain linolenic acid.

Gamma-linolenic is not found at all in either sunflower seed oil or safflower seed oil. In fact, it is only commercially available in the oil of the evening primrose.

Overall, evening primrose oil contains a higher percentage of essential fatty acids. The approximate figures are:

Evening Primrose: 80 per cent
Sunflower: 60 per cent
Safflower: 70 per cent

Table 1. Comparisons of Evening Primrose Oil with Sunflower Seed Oil and Safflower Seed Oil

Constituents	Evening Primrose (% Content)	Sunflower (% Content)	Safflower (% Content)
Gamma-linolenic	7-8	Nil	Nil
Linoleic	72	60	70
Palmitic	6	8	8
Stearic	2	4	2
Oleic	11	26	16

Evening primrose oil in capsule form is also easier to take than seed oils, which can be messy and can make you put on weight.

How to Buy Evening Primrose Oil Capsules
There are two major British manufacturers.

Naudicelle
Manufactured by:
    Bio-Oil Research Ltd.
    Royal Oak Building
    High Street
    CREWE
    Cheshire CW2 7BL
    England
    (Tel: 0270-213094)

Efamol G
Manufactured by:
    Efamol Ltd.
    40 Warton Road
    Stratford
    LONDON E15
    England
    (Tel: 01-555 9042)

Evening primrose oil capsules are also available in the following countries:

Canada
Efamol is available from:
    Primrose Research Inc.,
    Suite 11, 245 Victoria Avenue,
    Westmount, Montreal,
    P.Q. H3Z 2 M6

Denmark
Naudicelle is available from:
    Westag,
    Kurt West Agenturer,
    Baekvaj 13,
    Sdr. Vorupor,
    DL 7700 Thisted.

Norway
Naudicelle is available from:
    Mr J.A. Nystedt,
    Bioplant,
    Thv. Meyersgt 33,
    Oslo 5.

South Africa
Efamol is available from:
    Peppina Sales Co. (Pty) Ltd.,
    P.O. Box 9731,
    Johannesburg 2000.

Sweden
Pre-Glandin (the same as *Efamol G*) is available from:
    Sjostedt Intermedica Nordic AB,
    Banehagsgatan 1,
    Uppgang 7,
    S – 414 – 51,
    Goteborg.
Note: This agent for *Efamol* serves the whole of Scandinavia.

Naudicelle is available from:
    Mr C. Johansson,
    Brankato AB,
    Box 9105,
    (Besoksadr. Kantyxegatan 5),
    200 39 Malmo.

United States of America
Gamma Prim (the same as *Efamol G*) is available from any General Nutrition Corp. food store.

    Evening primrose oil capsules will shortly be available in some other countries. Write to the head office of Bio-Oil Research and Efamol Ltd. in England for details.

Toxicity Studies

These products have been subjected to extensive toxicity tests to the standards recommended by the U.K. Pharmaceutical Committee on the Toxicity and Safety of Drugs, and Product Licences have been granted by the United Kingdom Ministry of Health Licensing Authority.

However, despite rigorous campaigning, they are not available on the National Health Service in the U.K. However, there is nothing to stop you from buying them privately. They are at the moment classified as a food by the U.K. Borderline Substances Committee.

Vitamin F and Gamma
Evening primrose oil capsules are also sold commercially by mail order and in health food shops in Britain as *F-500* and *Gamma*.

How to Take Evening Primrose Oil Capsules

The dosage currently recommended is six capsules a day. Take two, three times a day, with meals. Swallow with water. Very few people report any side-effects at all. Some have noticed a loosening of the bowels. However, anyone with constipation would see this as a bonus. If diarrhoea is a problem when you first start taking the capsules, begin with only two capsules a day, and build up gradually to six as your body gets used to them.

What to Take with Evening Primrose Oil Capsules

(See Chapter 9 on vitamins and minerals.)

To work most efficiently, evening primrose oil capsules should be taken together with the following vitamins and minerals:

—— Vitamin E. This is essential to prevent the oxidation of unsaturated fats into dangerous peroxides. It also helps stabilize the E.F.A.s in the oil.
—— Vitamin C. Also acts as an anti-oxidant, and helps the conversion process of dihomo-gamma-linolenic acid to prostaglandins.
—— Vitamin B6. Necessary for the first stages of the biochemical conversion process of essential fatty acids.

—— Vitamin B3. Also necessary for the biochemical conversion process.

—— Zinc. Essential for the biochemical conversion process.

Note

If essential fatty acids are taken without vitamin E, they can be converted into peroxides and other substances which can be highly toxic. These substances may cause demyelination. Vitamin E has already been added to *Naudicelle* and *Efamol G* and they are, therefore, entirely safe to take on their own.

Foods to Avoid with Evening Primrose Oil Capsules

Avoid all foods high in saturated fats: fatty meats; milk; butter; cheese; cream; cakes and biscuits; processed foods made with palm oil or coconut oil. Foods rich in saturated fats have the effect of cancelling out the capsules. Excess saturated fat in the diet competes with essential fatty acids, and worsens the effect of an E.F.A. deficiency.

If you cannot avoid eating animal fats at a meal, like at a dinner party, take a couple of evening primrose oil capsules after the meal.

Reported Benefits

During 1979, a survey was carried out to assess the views of M.S. patients taking *Naudicelle* as a dietary supplement. 480 M.S. sufferers took part in the survey. Of these, 65 per cent felt there was some improvement in their condition. Of these, 43 per cent said there had been a stabilization of their condition – they had got no better, but they had got no worse. 22 per cent said there had been fewer and less severe attacks. 20 per cent said certain symptoms had been alleviated. 13 per cent reported an improvement in general health. 2 per cent reported further beneficial side-effects. The full results look like this:

Some improvement:	65 per cent
No change:	22 per cent
Deteriorated:	10 per cent
Don't know:	3 per cent

Improvements

People in the 'some improvement' category mentioned the following benefits:

—— Increased mobility.
—— Increased walking ability.
—— Reduced spasm or tremor.
—— Improved bladder function.
—— Improved eyesight.
—— Improved condition of hair and skin.
—— Relief of constipation.
—— Improvement in wound healing.
—— A lowering of cholesterol levels.
—— Regaining correct weight.
—— Heavy periods returned to normal.

Note. The 'improved' group contained a significantly higher proportion of M.S. patients who had been diagnosed within the preceding four years.

The ARMS Survey

In 1977 ARMS sent out a questionnaire to all its members to find out what effect *Naudicelle* was having on them. They were also asked to get an opinion from their own G.P. as to their condition since taking these capsules. 177 completed questionnaires were returned. These were the results:

Improved: 127
No change: 33
Worse: 17

Of the 127 in the 'improved' category, there were 59 testimonials from G.P.s supporting this assessment. (But not everybody who filled in the questionnaire bothered to see their doctor.)

Even though this survey has no scientific standing, and all the answers are based only on a subjective opinion of the M.S. person who filled in the questionnaire, the results are nevertheless extremely encouraging.

Length of Time Taking Capsules

ARMS members were also asked how long they had been

taking *Naudicelle*. The answers showed that improvements increased when they had been taking the capsules for more than four months. Beneficial effects appeared as follows:

Under 4 months:	35 per cent
4 months–1 year:	73 per cent
1-2 years:	73 per cent
2-3 years:	82 per cent

At the time of the survey, very few members had been on *Naudicelle* for longer than three years.

Diet
141 of the people who returned completed questionnaires were also on some kind of diet. The results showed that the people who were exercising some control over what they ate said that *Naudicelle* had beneficial results, more than those who were not on any diet.

Other Surveys on Evening Primrose Oil
Unfortunately, other surveys have not shown such encouraging results. One other study found that:

15-20 per cent may be helped in a major way.
15-20 per cent may be helped in a minor way.
60-70 per cent may not be helped at all.

How do you know whether you are one of the lucky ones who can experience dramatic improvements? The only way is to try for yourself and see; but you must give it time. It takes about six to twelve weeks for the red blood cells to show any difference, but probably several months before you actually notice any real improvement. So do not give up if nothing happens straight away. You must be patient.

It is only honest to add that there have been other trials in which no clear beneficial results have been shown with *Naudicelle* on M.S. patients. However, critics of these trials point out that there was no check on the diet of patients on the trials. It is known that a diet high in animal fat inhibits the effect of these capsules, and there was nothing to stop the patients eating whatever they liked.

Also, *Naudicelle* used to be sold in capsules which were coated with a distinctive black and orange dye. It has since been found that this dye inhibited the conversion process.

Both *Naudicelle* and *Efamol G* now come in a clear edible gelatin capsule, which does not inhibit the conversion process.

Note. All these trials took place before *Efamol G* was available on the market. The results for *Efamol G* should be taken as the same as those for *Naudicelle*.

Testimonials

Written tributes to *Naudicelle* have been arriving in substantial numbers through Joe Osborne's letter-box. He has collected many of these in his book, *A Guide To The Management of Multiple Sclerosis: Naudicelle, Dietary, Exercise* (see *Further Reading*).

It should be noted that the old black-and-orange capsules appear on the cover. *Naudicelle* capsules do *not* look like this any longer. Further, since that book was published, *Efamol G* has come onto the market.

5   DIET

There has been some very interesting detective work going on into the possible link between geographical areas and M.S. Scientists call this epidemiology. In general, studies show that M.S. is highest where people eat a lot of animal fats, and lowest where they do not.

Also, M.S. has been on the increase since a change in diet. The high standard of living has meant that most people in the West have been eating more meat, butter, cheese and other dairy produce, plus more processed, refined and tinned foods. In the last sixty years or so, there has been a significant increase in the consumption of processed and hardened vegetable oils, such as hard margarine.

The 'Beer-Butter' Countries
If you look at a map of the world, you will see that the geographical distribution of M.S. falls broadly into the same areas where there is a 'beer-butter' culture. These are the countries – or parts of countries – which have a high content of animal fat in their diet. The countries include the British Isles, Scandinavia, Holland, Belgium, Germany, northern France, northern Switzerland, U.S.A., Canada, Australia and New Zealand.

The fact that beer is popular in these areas probably has more to do with the culture, rather than being directly related to M.S.

The 'Wine-Oil' Countries

There is a low incidence of M.S. where the diet is lower in animal fats, and higher in vegetable oils and fish.

These countries include Spain, Italy, southern France, southern Switzerland, Greece, parts of the Middle East, and North Africa.

The Distribution of M.S. Within One Country

There have been some very interesting studies which have investigated the geographical distribution of M.S. within one country. The most notable have been comparisons between the Orkneys and Shetland Isles in Scotland, north and south Switzerland, and the coastal and inland areas of Norway.

Similar facts emerged from all three studies: M.S. was higher in the areas of dairy farming, where the population ate a lot of animal fat, and lower in the areas where people ate less animal produce but more fish.

In Norway, for example, there were nearly four times as many cases of M.S. inland where there is dairy farming, than along the coast, where they eat a lot of fish.

These are simply clues. No one has confirmed in a scientific trial that these factors are decisive in M.S. Scientists involved in nutrition have, however, found these facts sufficiently startling to use them as a partial basis for diet therapy for M.S.

The Relationship Between Fats and Multiple Sclerosis

Quite apart from the geographical clues to M.S., there have been a lot of studies connecting M.S. with fats. Research has shown that people with M.S. seem to have something wrong with their ability to handle fats. They are deficient in the essential fatty acids, and the biochemical conversion processes in the body are not working efficiently at turning some of the food you eat into the various end-products which your nervous system needs.

There have also been studies to show that people with M.S. have adverse effects when they eat meals high in animal fat. Tests have shown that the red blood cells clump together after a high fat meal. When this happens, the circulation slows down, and there is a reduced supply of oxygen to the tissues. This affects the brain, heart and other organs.

Another theory suggests that M.S. people might have an inability to metabolize large amounts of saturated fats.

The geographical distribution of M.S. and its relationship to diet, plus the knowledge scientists have on the role of essential fatty acids in M.S., have been the basis for two dietary regimes for M.S. sufferers.

One, known as the 'Swank Low Fat Diet', was formulated more than thirty years ago in Canada by an American neurologist, Professor Roy Swank.

The second was formulated by Dr Michael Crawford, a bio-chemist at the Nuffield Laboratories of Comparative Medicine in London, who has done a lot of research into essential fatty acids. The dietary regime which he recommends has been used widely by members of ARMS (Action for Research into Multiple Sclerosis).

THE SWANK LOW-FAT DIET

—— Essential oils (see list below) must be included in the quantity of at least 20g (4 teaspoonful) a day.
—— Fat in meat, poultry, liver and eggs must be kept down to 15g (3 teaspoonful) a day.
—— Fat-containing red meats should be eaten only two days a week.
—— Complete banning of all dairy products, and all processed foods containing hidden fat, (see list).

Foods Containing the Essential Fatty Acids

Take a minimum of 4 teaspoonful a day of essential oils. Working, walking people could well increase their essential oil intake to 8 teaspoonful. Very active people could take 10 teaspoonful.

Vegetable Oils

Sunflower seed oil
Safflower seed oil
Soybean oil
Peanut oil

Corn oil
Olive oil
Linseed oil

Note. Professor Swank developed his diet before evening primrose oil came on the market; but you can safely add it to this list.

Fish Oils
Cod liver oil
Tuna fish
Salmon
Sardines
Herring
Mackerel

Nuts and Seeds
Sunflower seeds
Sesame seeds
Peanuts (and peanut butter as long as non-hydrogenated)
Almonds
Cashews

Vegetables
Dark green leafy vegetables contain E.F.A.s of the alpha-linolenic family, especially spinach.

Foods Allowed in Any Quantity
These foods contain none, or very little, saturated fat.

Eggs, whites only.
White fish, any kind.
Shellfish, any kind.
Breast of poultry with skin removed.
Skimmed milk; powdered skimmed milk; buttermilk.
Rinsed low-fat cottage cheese.
Yogurt made with skimmed milk.
99 per cent fat-free cheese.
Clear soups: beef or chicken broth; *bouillon; consommé.*
Wholemeal bread.
Matzos.
Whole grain cereals.
Rice.

Pasta.
Corn meal.
All fresh fruit.
All fresh vegetables (cook vegetables with steamer or eat raw).
Frozen or canned vegetables without butter.
Jam and marmalade.
Honey.
Sugar, molasses, treacle, maple syrup.
Jelly.
Tea, coffee.
Carbonated and alcoholic drinks in moderation.

Note. Soft, polyunsaturated margarines were not available in the U.S.A. when this diet was compiled. However, there are many soft margarines in the U.K. which can safely be added to this list (e.g. *Flora*).

Moderately Allowed Saturated Fat Foods

Eat only 3 teaspoonsful of fat a day, maximum. The largest single source of fat in our diet is meat.

Table 2. Fat Content of Food

Food	Amount equal to 1 teaspoonful of fat
Eggs	1 whole
Chicken gizzards	3 oz
Chicken livers	3 oz
Heart: calf, beef	3 oz
Kidney: pork, veal, lamb	3 oz
Leg of lamb	3 oz
Liver: beef, calf or pork	3 oz
Tongue: calf	3 oz
Venison	3 oz

Table 2. *continued*

Food	Amount equal to 1 teaspoonful of fat
Beef, lean	2 oz
Chicken and turkey – dark meat, skin removed	2 oz
Chicken and turkey hearts	2 oz
Heart: lamb	2 oz
Ham, lean	2 oz
Kidney: beef	2 oz
Lamb: rib, loin, shoulder	2 oz
Pheasant, skin removed	2 oz
Pork, lean	2 oz
Rabbit	2 oz
Tongue: beef	2 oz
Veal	2 oz
Bacon	1 oz
Duck	1 oz

Forbidden Foods

Dairy Products
Whole milk; cream; butter; sour cream; ice cream; natural and processed cheese of any kind; all imitation dairy products (often contain palm oil which is saturated fat).

Fats and Oils
All hard margarines; shortening; lard; chocolate; cocoa butter; coconut; coconut and palm oils.

Packet Foods
All packaged commercial mixes for cakes, biscuits etc. Potato crisps; party-type snacks.

Processed Meat and Poultry
Luncheon meat; salami; frankfurters; all sausages; canned meat products.

Pastries
All commercially-prepared pies, cakes, pastries, doughnuts, biscuits.

Tinned Foods
Containing cream (e.g. cream soups); meat; or dairy produce.

Food Supplements

—— Vitamin E can be taken in capsules, as wheatgerm, or as wheatgerm oil to act as an anti-oxidant.
—— One teaspoonful of cod liver oil a day, or cod liver oil capsules (6 to 8 a day). This provides E.F.A.s of the alpha-linolenic family.
—— A multi-vitamin and mineral capsule. (See Chapter 9 on Vitamins and Minerals.)

General Guidelines to the Swank Low-fat Diet
Ideally, eat fresh foods. If you have to buy tinned or packet foods, read the label carefully. If any product does not specify the kind of vegetable oil used, avoid it. Weigh food after it has been cooked, not before. Use only whole grain products (wholemeal bread, brown rice, wholewheat spaghetti etc.).

Protein Intake
Although this is not a vegetarian diet, most protein should be taken from foods other than red meat. At least five days a week, you should get your protein from eggs, fish, seafood, skinned chicken or turkey breast. Fish contains as much protein and amino acids as meat, and is an important part of this diet.

Quantities
The fat and oil intake should be distributed over the course of the day. Eat three or four meals of about the same size, instead of snacks here and there, and a heavy meal at the end of the day.

Eating Out
Avoid creamed foods, gravies, sauces. Avoid fried foods,

including chips (re-heated oil becomes like saturated fat). Avoid butter and cream, and foods cooked in them. Avoid puddings, except fruit salad.

Chinese and Japanese food is generally low in saturated fat and high in unsaturated fat. (Except spare ribs, duck, and deep-fried dishes.)

If you are asked out to a dinner party, it is wise to warn the hostess in advance about your diet.

Alcohol

Allowed in small quantities. (But see Chapter 10 on Drinking and Smoking.)

Rest

Professor Swank recommends that his low-fat diet is combined with adequate rest. Physical and mental fatigue must be avoided. Patients are instructed to rest a minimum of one hour a day, ideally lying down after lunch. (See Chapter 12 on Fatigue.)

Note: Since Professor Swank wrote his book he has made some slight modifications to his diet. Now he allows NO RED MEAT (beef, pork or lamb) during the first year. After that, he allows only 100g twice a week. He publishes regular newsletters about his diet obtainable from the University of Oregon, Health Sciences Center, Portland, Oregan 97201, U.S.A.

Success of the Swank Low-fat Diet

Professor Swank claims a remarkable success rate. He says that 90-95 per cent of patients who began his diet in the early stages of M.S., with little or no evident disability, did not get worse during thirty years on the diet.*

Patients who started the diet later in the course of the disease, with definite disability, did get worse, but at a much slower rate than normal. In a few cases their condition stabilized.

He says his diet prolongs active, productive life. Patients got stronger, and remained energetic, stable, and attack-free. Old

---

* For further information on the Swank Low-fat Diet see *The Multiple Sclerosis Diet Book* by Professor Roy L. Swank (Doubleday, New York). Available in the U.K. from ARMS, 71 Gray's Inn Road, London WC1X 8TR.).

signs and symptoms may still have been there, but new ones
rarely developed.

Patients who started the diet after becoming disabled noted
an increased feeling of well-being. Most patients had fewer
colds and tummy upsets, and noted an increase in energy.
There was a 95 per cent reduction in the frequency of attacks,
and the attacks that did happen were mild, infrequent and
brief.

Professor Swank found that patients on the low-fat diet
were able to work and walk for longer. Over 10 years, about 50
per cent of M.S. people on no diet at all who could walk and
work at the beginning could not do so at the end of 10 years.
Whereas only 25 per cent of Swank's patients, all on the low-
fat diet, could not work or walk after 10 years.

Death-rates are lower too. M.S. people not on the diet died
at the rate of 20-28 per cent at the end of a 15-year research
study. Whereas only 6 per cent of the low-fat diet M.S.
patients died in the same period.

After a 30-year research period, 63 per cent of M.S. people
not on the low-fat diet had died, and 18 per cent of the M.S.
people who had been on the low-fat diet the whole time, had
died.

This means that the average reduction of the death rate
among M.S. people on the low-fat diet is two-thirds to three-
quarters the normal death rate for M.S. sufferers.

THE ESSENTIAL FATTY ACID DIET

This diet has become familiarly known by ARMS members in
England as the 'Dr Crawford Diet', because it was Dr Michael
Crawford, of the Nuffield Laboratories of Comparative
Medicine in London who formulated this nutritional
approach to M.S. He is now on the management committee of
the ARMS Unit at the Central Middlesex Hospital, and is in
charge of the nutritional management of the people with M.S.
who go to the unit. This is the diet they will be given. It has
been used by ARMS members enthusiastically for several
years.

The Thinking Behind This Diet

The rationale for this diet is partly based on the geographical
distribution of M.S. (see page 41). M.S. is low in areas where
the population eats a lot of food rich in alpha-linolenic acid

and its derivatives, such as fish.

Another basis for this diet is that the brains of people with M.S. are deficient in essential fatty acids. This structural deficiency probably happened at a very early age, and this inadequate structure of E.F.A.s in the brain means that when something happens (e.g. a viral infection?) it is susceptible, and cannot withstand the attack.

An additional reason for focusing on an E.F.A. diet is that 60 per cent of the solid matter of the brain and 70 per cent of the myelin sheath is lipids (fats).

The essential fatty acid component of the brain is dominated by the long-chain derivatives of linoleic acids and alpha-linolenic acids, and this diet concentrates on foods rich in arachidonic acid and cervonic acid.

Also, the blood of people with M.S. is known to have low levels of E.F.A.s. However, this is not specific to M.S., and may be part of having any chronic disease.

All these factors are connected with nutrition because the only way the body can get the E.F.A.s is by eating the foods that contain them.

The Aim of the Essential Fatty Acid Diet

The aim of the Essential Fatty Acid Diet is to correct the deficiencies in the structure of the central nervous system, and the function of the immune system. It has been shown that changes in the blood plasma of M.S. people on this diet happen very quickly, though it can take between nine months and a year for the red blood cells to be corrected. It seems possible that the chemical structure of the central nervous system can be corrected by diet.

Whether it is possible to correct the function of the central nervous system is less certain. The ultimate goal of this diet would be to activate whatever it is that is happening in the body when someone with M.S. is in a remission. But, as well as being a remission agent, the aim of this diet is to defend the body against attack.

This diet concentrates on E.F.A.s because they are the building blocks of the central nervous system. It avoids saturated fats because they cancel out the good effects of E.F.A.s. Yet, this diet also provides all the nutrients needed for health, such as proteins, carbohydrates, vitamins and minerals. It is an extremely healthy diet, and would be good and easy to follow for every member of the family, not just the person with M.S.

Some General Rules

1. Eat at least ½ lb (225g) of liver each week (rich in arachidonic acid).
2. Eat at least three fish meals a week (rich in cervonic acid).
3. Eat a large helping of dark green vegetables daily, e.g. spinach or greens (alpha-linolenic acid).
4. Eat some raw vegetables daily, as a salad, with dressing made with a seed oil.
5. Eat some linseeds, or cod liver oil daily (alpha-linolenic acid).
6. Eat some fresh fruit daily.
7. Eat as much fresh food as possible, in preference to processed food.
8. Choose lean cuts of meat. Trim all fat off meat before cooking.
9. Avoid hard animal fats like butter, lard, suet, dripping, and foods high in saturated fats such as cream, cheese etc.
10. Eat whole grain cereals and wholemeal bread rather than the refined versions.
11. Cut down on sugar and dishes containing sugar.

Foods to Eat

Meat
Lean meat is a good source of arachidonic acid, particularly wild or game meats like partridge, venison, pigeon, etc. These do not have the fattiness of animals reared for intensive farming. However, more ordinary lean meat is acceptable. Go for lean pork, gammon, beef, lamb, chicken, turkey, and rabbit. Trim all the visible fat away from the meat before cooking it, as the fat is saturated fat and to be avoided. Do not eat the skin of chicken or turkey.

Offal
Offal is the organ meats: liver, kidneys, brains, sweetbreads. Offal is particularly rich in arachidonic acid. Liver is the best source, so aim to eat at least ½ lb (225g) of fresh liver (any

kind) a week. Dried or dessicated liver tablets have lost much
of the goodness of fresh liver.

Fish

Marine foods are the richest source of cervonic acid, an
essential nutrient for the brain. Eat at least three fish meals a
week. Any freshwater fish, marine fish, or shellfish is fine.
Choose from mackerel, trout, tuna, crab, lobster, salmon,
sardines, mussels, cod roe, herring, sprats, whitebait, squid,
prawns, shrimps, cod, plaice, haddock, all white fish, etc.
Fresh fish is best, and frozen second-best. Tinned fish (e.g.
sardines, tuna) is very much third-best. Fish can be cooked
any way you like, except in butter. Fish deep-fried at the fish
and chip shop is likely to be saturated in saturated fat.

Fruit and Vegetables

Eat plenty of fresh fruit and vegetables. All vegetables are
good, but the greener the vegetable the better as they are an
excellent source of alpha-linolenic acid, e.g. spinach, broccoli,
kale, green pepper, parsley, green beans. Eat a large helping
of one or two of these vegetables daily. Germinal vegetables
like beansprouts are very good too.

The coloured vegetables (e.g. tomatoes, carrots, beetroot,
red peppers, red cabbage), apart from being rich in vitamins
and minerals, help prevent the oxidation of E.F.A.s, because
of their vitamin C and E content. They 'mop up' the free
oxygen. So you should eat a salad every day for lunch, ideally
made with a dressing made with sunflower seed oil or
safflower seed oil, or one of the other seed oils.

All other vegetables (e.g. potatoes, turnips, mushrooms) are
good too and help to make interesting recipes when used with
the key foods.

Frozen fruit and vegetables are an acceptable second-best to
fresh ones.

Pulses

These include peas, beans, lentils etc. These are good sources
of alpha-linolenic acid and protein, and are good in salads.

Nuts

A good source of E.F.A.s. Make sure that peanut butter is
pure and natural and not hydrogenated.

Seeds, Seed Oils and Other Oils

The best oils to cook with are sunflower seed oil, safflower seed oil, olive oil, corn oil, soya bean oil, or sesame seed oil. These all contain linoleic acid, and soya bean oil also contains alpha-linolenic acid.

Avoid blends of unnamed vegetable oils, and whichever oil you use, do not heat it to the point of smoking, and do not use it more than once. Throw it away after one use. This is because overheating and exposure to air damages the E.F.A. activity. Once opened, keep your oil in the fridge. To get the full benefit of these oils, it is best to take them uncooked, as a salad dressing.

Use polyunsaturated soft margarines (e.g. *Flora*) for spreading on bread and for baking.

Seeds can be eaten on their own. Sunflower seeds and sesame seeds are obtainable from health food shops. Linseeds are an excellent source of alpha-linolenic acid, and are obtainable either from health food shops, or seed merchants. *Linusit Gold*, which is split linseeds, is more palatable and can be sprinkled on breakfast cereals.

The seed oil richest in E.F.A.s is evening primrose oil, which can only be taken in capsule form. (See Chapter 4 on evening primrose.)

Bread and Cereals

Unrefined cereals and wholemeal bread are fine. As well as containing the germ, which contains E.F.A.s and vitamins, whole cereals also include the husk of the grain which provides bulk and helps bowel action. This is because bran has a high roughage content. Wholewheat pasta is also fine.

Other Acceptable Foods

Any whole, natural foods are fine, for example: pure honey; brown rice; raw sugar; eggs. The white of an egg contains no fat. The yolk contains a mixture of saturated and unsaturated fats. Provided you do not have more than three or four eggs a week, they can be included in the diet. Seasonings, herbs and spices are also acceptable.

Reduced-intake foods

Dairy Produce
The fat in milk is almost all saturated, with only about 3 per cent of the fatty acids polyunsaturated. Skimmed milk, with the cream taken off, is acceptable, but dried skimmed milk in tins should be avoided, as should any skimmed milk with added vegetable fat. Also, low-fat yogurt is fine. Cottage cheese made from low-fat (skimmed milk) is fine too.

Foods Made with Sugar
High nutrient foods should always be eaten in preference to filling foods with empty calories. So cut down on sugary foods.

Foods to Avoid
High-fat dairy produce and anything made with butter, cream, or hard cheeses.

Manufactured meat products, e.g. spam, luncheon meat, *patés*, pastes, pork pies and other shop-bought meat pies, sausages, hamburgers. Shop-bought cakes, biscuits and pastries will contain a lot of saturated fat.

Also avoid refined cereal products.

Recipes and Menus
Judith Harding, the nutritionist at the ARMS Unit at the Central Middlesex Hospital, has compiled a list of recipes based on the essential fatty acid diet.

She has specially designed many recipes for people who do not much like liver and other offal, and fish. These include such tasty treats as 'Liver Provençale'. She guarantees that you will like liver and fish once you have tried her recipes. Available from:

ARMS/CPG Unit
Central Middlesex Hospital
Acton Lane
Park Royal
LONDON NW10 7NS
(Tel. 01-961 4911)

DR PAUL EVERS' DIET

Dr Evers runs a clinic in West Germany concentrating on treating M.S. patients with a special diet. It has certain similarities to the previous two diets, and some specific differences. Like the other diets, he emphasizes the importance of essential fatty acids in the diet, and prefers vegetable foods to animal foods. On the other hand, he does allow milk, milk products, cheese, and eggs, as long as they are farm-fresh.

Some people have given some very glowing reports about Dr Evers' diet. It contains very healthy advice, although some people might find it a rather acquired taste. It certainly has a Germanic flavour about it.

The Basics

—— Vegetable foods should be eaten in preference to animal foods.

—— More than half the fats eaten should be polyunsaturated and unsaturated fatty acids.

—— Avoid a high calorie intake.

Recommended Foods

Raw fruits, fresh and dried.
Grains, whole.
Nuts, fresh and untreated.
Raw vegetables, including root crops.
Whole grain bread.
Honey, natural.
Eggs, fresh, free-range.
Milk and milk products – direct from healthy, grazing animals.
Cheeses – all natural varieties, including quark made without salt and sugar.
Butter, farm-made.
Vegetable oils – sunflower seed, safflower seed, wheatgerm oil, maize germ oil.

At a later stage, when there has been an improvement, more foods are added to the diet:

Smoked meat.
Fresh salmon.
Raw ham.
Raw lean meat.
Freshwater fish – steamed or lightly fried, in seed oils.
Game.
Poultry.
All herbs.

The key to the choice of all foods is leave the food as natural as possible, and eat it as fresh as possible.

Chew fruit and root vegetables well, or grate them. Raw foods should be eaten in preference to cooked foods. Combine raw root vegetables and fruit in salads.

Table 3. Recommended Average Daily Amounts

Food	Amounts
Germinated grain	50-100g (2-4 oz)
Whole grain bread	Up to about 200g (7 oz)
Rolled oats	70g (3 oz) or more
Fruit and vegetables	450g (1 lb) or more
Milk	1 litre (about 2 pints) or more
Butter	30g (1 oz) or more
Honey	As desired
Linseeds, sunflower seeds, nuts	120g (just over 4 oz)
One egg	

Foods to Avoid

Refined carbohydrates, e.g. white sugar, sweets, refined white flour, cakes, biscuits, pastries.
Chocolate.
Preserved and tinned foods.
All highly spiced foods.
Mustard.
Vinegar.
Saccharin.
Coffee.
Cigarettes (absolutely banned).

Constipation

If you follow this diet correctly, there should be no problems with constipation and you should be regular. However, if you do get constipated: chew fresh whole fruit, and before each meal take linseeds or soaked prunes.

Drink
For special occasions, a glass of wine or beer is allowed. Dr Evers recommends milk with meals.

Germinated Grain
This is when the grain begins to sprout little green shoots. It can be done with wheat, available from health food shops, or a variety of grains which are sold in packets with instructions for sprouting (alfalfa etc.).

To Sprout Wheat
1. Put the grain in a dish (or several dishes) of water, in the evening.
2. In the morning, drain the water.
3. During the day, leave the grain covered with a cloth.
4. In the evening, pour water over the grain. The grain should be rinsed in the morning, midday and in the evenings in a sieve.
5. In 3-5 days a small green sprout begins to appear from each grain.
6. Eat it at this stage.
7. The grain should be eaten fresh daily.
8. Keep several dishes going at once, at different stages so you always have a fresh supply.

Recipes
Dr Evers has written a short booklet called: *Help Fight M.S. – Dietary Therapy with Polyunsaturated Fatty Acids*. (From Klinik Dr Evers, 5768 Sundern-Langscheid, West Germany.)

6 THE EXCLUSION DIETS

The diets in the previous chapter are firmly based on the importance of essential fatty acids for the central nervous system. The diets in this chapter are based more on what could be called the 'food allergy principle', i.e. that people with M.S. are for some reason allergic to certain foods. The theory, put very simply, is that the patient improves if certain foods are excluded from the diet, and gets worse if they continue to eat them.

The most well-known diet in this category is the Gluten-Free Diet developed by British playwright Roger MacDougall, and which underwent various modifications during the 1970s.

The other well-publicized one is known as 'The Rita Greer Diet'. Rita Greer painstakingly worked out this diet for her husband Alan, who had a particularly severe case of M.S., but has now regenerated to the point where he can run and climb ladders. This diet includes many of the principles of the essential fatty acid diets, but it is primarily an exclusion diet based on allergy to particular foods.

Food Allergies and M.S.

The connection between food allergies and M.S. has not been put to any sort of scientific trial. Yet there are plenty of people with M.S. who will testify that they became allergic to certain foods only after M.S. was diagnosed. This allergy did not exist before the onset of M.S. This may be part of the disease process showing that the immune system has gone wrong, rather than a cause of the disease. However, no one knows for sure.

The problem with any diet based on food allergies is that one person with M.S. may be allergic to a particular food, but the next person with M.S. may not be. They may be allergic to something completely different.

On the other hand, many people with M.S. have religiously kept to either the Gluten-Free Diet or the Rita Greer Diet, and have felt wonderful for it. In their case, it may be that they are allergic to the same foods as Roger MacDougall or Alan Greer, but there are also many people who have been on these diets who have noticed no difference in their condition.

The only sure way to find out what foods you personally are allergic to is to laboriously test each one. For that reason I am including a section on testing foods for allergic reactions at the end of this chapter.

ROGER MACDOUGALL'S DIET:
THE GLUTEN-FREE PLUS DIET

Roger MacDougall's diet is popularly known as the Gluten-Free Diet, but it has undergone many modifications since its early days and now includes four equally important elements:

1. No gluten.
2. Low refined sugar.
3. Low saturated fats.
4. Mineral and vitamin supplements.

This diet has many similarities with Rita Greer's diet (which came many years later). Both were discovered by one lay person using a process of inspiration coupled with arduous trial and error. In both cases the diets have had a remarkable regenerative effect on the individuals for whom the diets were designed.

The other similarities between the two diets are that both

exclude gluten, sugar, and saturated fats and supplement the diet with vitamins and minerals. The Roger MacDougall diet does not go as far as the Rita Greer diet in excluding certain other foods.

The Theory of Roger MacDougall

Roger MacDougall, like Alan Greer, has a startling story to tell. He is now 70 and is jetting round the world, writing and lecturing, and is in good health with no signs of disability. Yet in 1953 he was firmly diagnosed as having M.S. and showed many of the classic symptoms. Within a few years of diagnosis his eyesight, legs, fingers and speech were badly affected. Before long, he was in a wheelchair.

Without any medical training (he is a playwright and professor in the University of California's theatre department), Roger MacDougall decided to set about finding ways of treating his degenerative condition. He hit upon treating M.S. in the same way as Coeliac disease, where the patient is allergic to gluten.

The reasons why Roger MacDougall linked M.S. with coeliac disease is because in coeliac disease the patient cannot assimilate fats. However, once wheat, barley, oats and rye are removed totally from the diet, fats can be taken into the body without any problem. MacDougall suggests that foods containing gluten 'damage the lining of the small intestine in such a way that the nutrients required to keep renewing the myelin sheath are prevented from reaching the bloodstream'.

As another explanation, he says, 'perhaps the gluten amalgamates with the necessary nutrients during the course of digestion in such a way that they are carried down with other waste matter and therefore do not become available'. Another possibility he puts forward is 'that gluten attacks not only the mucous lining of the intestine ... but also many similar tissues in other parts of the body, and that this gives rise to other degenerative conditions'.

Roger MacDougall's theory goes on to suggest that gluten, excessive animal fat, and refined sugar are things which have been added to our diet since the development of agriculture and are in fact alien to our metabolism.

This diet has not been put to any strict scientific trial, though recently researchers from the National Institute of Mental Health in Washington found that gluten gives rise to substances called opioids in the gut. Some people cannot digest these, and researchers have found that they block the conversion of dihomo-gamma-linolenic acid to prostaglandins series 1.

An Australian doctor, Dr R. Shatin from Melbourne, has suggested that the demyelination of the nerve sheaths is secondary to an intolerance of gluten in the small intestine. He also put forward the hypothesis that the high rate of M.S. in Canada, Scotland and Western Ireland may be due to the predominating use of Canadian wheat, which has the highest content of gluten of any in the world.

The best most doctors have to say about Roger MacDougall's diet is that it cannot do you any harm. However, there are thousands of people who have stuck to Roger MacDougall's diet who will testify to its benefits and can show you how their condition has improved. On the other hand, there are many thousands who have stuck to the diet for a short time and then given it up because they could not see any improvements at all.

Roger MacDougall used himself as a guinea pig, and he says it took him all of fifteen years to recover to the point where he could run about and stand on one leg. He says he has not suffered a relapse the entire time he has been on his diet. Because he knows it can take years to show any significant effects, he urges patience, to give it time to work. He emphatically does not claim this diet is a *cure* for M.S., but a way of controlling the disease.

Excluded Foods

Grains
Exclude anything containing gluten: found in wheat, barley, oats, and rye. (Gluten is a protein found in these grains. It is the stuff that gives uncooked pastry its elasticity.) Do not eat anything made with these grains, for example: bread; cakes; biscuits; crispbreads; pasta; many breakfast cereals; vast numbers of tinned and processed foods (look on the label).

Sugar
No refined sugar, or any product containing it; for example: jams, marmalades, cakes, biscuits, tinned fruit, sweets, chocolate, ice cream, most drinks, processed foods, etc.

Saturated Fats
Cut out butter, cream, full cream milk, high-fat cheeses.

Meat
Do not eat fatty meats like bacon, pork, duck, goose, or processed meats like sausages, as they contain a lot of saturated fat.

Fruit and Vegetables
Cut out any tinned fruit and vegetables.

Flavourings and Condiments
Avoid anything with artificial colouring or flavouring.

Drinks
Many drinks contain either gluten or sugar or both. Give up ale, beer, whisky, gin, instant coffee, drinking chocolate, malted drinks, etc.

Foods You Can Eat

Cereals
Rice, maize (corn) and millet do not contain gluten. You can safely use products such as rice flour, cornflour, breakfast cereals made with rice and corn (with no added sugar); sago; tapioca.

Vegetables and Pulses
All vegetables and legumes, lightly cooked or raw. Pulses such as chick peas, butter beans, kidney beans etc. can be used as thickening agents and provide bulk.
   Potatoes should be cooked in their jackets. Chips should be fried in sunflower seed oil that is used only once and then thrown away.
   Salad vegetables should be eaten in large quantities, often. Eat a lot of dark green leafy vegetables and sprouting seeds, as they are rich in alpha-linolenic acid. It is best to eat fresh vegetables, though frozen will do.

Fats
Use only polyunsaturated margarine (e.g. *Flora*). For cooking and salad dressing, use sunflower seed oil or safflower seed oil.

Dairy Produce
You can use small quantities of skimmed milk; low-fat cottage cheese; low-fat yogurt; eggs.

Meat
Any offal is best: liver; kidneys; tongue; sweetbreads; brain; or any free-range animal such as venison, rabbit, poultry. Buy lean cuts of beef, pork etc.

Fish
You can eat any fish, fresh, frozen or tinned.

Sweet Things
Honey; raw Barbados sugar (not demerara); raw sugar chocolate; fructose.

Fruit and Nuts
All fruit and dried fruits. Can be fresh, frozen (but not tinned). All nuts acceptable.

Herbs, Spices, Condiments
All acceptable, but use only natural essences and flavourings. Use sodium-free salt, e.g. *Ruthmol*.

Drinks
Fruit and vegetable juices (natural and sugar-free); *Complan*; tea; decaffeinated coffee; cyder; *Babycham*; distilled water in preference to tap water.

Vitamin and Mineral Supplements
Roger MacDougall is involved in the marketing of a multi-vitamin and mineral tablet named, appropriately, *RM*. See Chapter 9 on vitamins and minerals for details. He also recommends daily doses of vitamin B12, which is particularly important for people who do not eat meat.

Roger MacDougall has written a booklet called *My Fight Against Multiple Sclerosis*. This, plus the *RM* supplements, can be obtained from:

Regenics Ltd.
25-27 Oxford Street
LONDON W1R 1RF
(Tel. 01-437 7651)

Recipes and Menus

Roger MacDougall himself has not devised any recipes or menus, but these have been invented very successfully by other people working along the same lines.

One excellent book is called *Good Food, Gluten-Free* by Hilda Cherry Hills (see *Further Reading*). The same firm also publishes a booklet called *Gluten-Free Diet: Optimum Gluten-Free Diet for Multiple Sclerosis*, also written by Hilda Cherry Hills. This includes a few recipes.

Mrs Hills objects strongly to the gluten-free flour on the market. She says:

> It is made from roller-milled bleached white flour, which means it has had its original minerals and vitamins drastically removed, and although there has been some addition of vitamin B1, niacin and iron, this only represents a small percentage of those taken out and there is no replacement of the vitamin E and the essential fatty acid, linoleic acid, which have been totally destroyed. Furthermore, it is frequently found so unpalatable (especially in bread) that the eater gives it up in disgust and returns to the ordinary gluten-containing bread which is toxic for him. This gluten-free flour has no therapeutic value.

As an alternative, she suggests rice flour bread. Rita Greer has come up with a more palatable gluten-free flour, and a ready-made gluten-free bread mix which makes passably good bread.

She has also written several good gluten-free, sugar-free, saturated-fat free cook books (see next section and *Further Reading*).

Rita Greer's and Hilda Cherry Hills' books can be obtained by mail order (also Rita Greer's foods and food mixes) from:

Cantassium Company,
225 Putney Bridge Road,
LONDON SW15 2PY

This company has also published its own booklet called *The Cantamac Dietary System*. This includes some recipes and is available free from the above address.

THE RITA GREER DIET

Rita Greer began experimenting with foods for her husband Alan at a time when he was severely disabled and doctors had written him off as a hopeless case. Her first breakthrough was when she accidentally discovered that Alan felt better on a diet which totally excluded meat – something she was forced to do through sheer poverty. From that, it was a short step to discover that he reacted badly to eggs and cheese, and all saturated fat.

Rita also decided to follow the principles of the Gluten-Free Diet, and cut out everything made with wheat, barley, oats and rye.

By this time, sunflower seed oil was gaining popularity as a supplement for M.S. patients. So she began by giving him large daily doses of sunflower seed oil. But as soon as *Naudicelle* became available she replaced the sunflower seed oil with these capsules of evening primrose oil.

With much trial and error, hard work, studying nutrition, and the creativity that goes with Rita being a gifted artist, she eventually came up with a diet that suited Alan's body perfectly.

She kept him on this basically vegan diet for about four years, during which time he made gigantic improvements to the point where the wheelchair and walking aids were banished with the bedpans to the lumber room.

His regeneration has been so startling that some doctors were doubtful how he could ever have been diagnosed as having M.S. at all, as his present condition does not tally with his medical notes. There is no doubt, however, that Alan Greer did and does have M.S. It is just that he now seems to have found the way of controlling the disease.

Neither Rita nor Alan Greer put this miraculous regeneration entirely down to the diet alone. The diet was used alongside other therapies, particularly exercise and leading a stress-free life.

This diet goes beyond the Gluten-Free Diet. It is totally Gluten-Free, but excludes many other items too.

Excluded Foods

Rita Greer had an easy task finding out which foods made Alan worse – he was sick if he ate something he was allergic to. This is a very dramatic response, and allergic reactions are usually more subtle (see section on testing for food allergies). The banned foods are as follows:

Dairy Products
Butter, cheese, milk, cream, yogurt, lard, eggs.

Meat/Fish
Meat, fatty fish like herring and tuna, shellfish.

Cereals
Wheat, barley, oats, rye and everything made with them –
bread, pasta, biscuits, cakes, breakfast cereals, custard
powder.

Sweets
Cane sugar, honey, jam, treacle, sweets, chocolate.

Drinks
Drinking chocolate, malted drinks, cocoa, coffee, strong tea,
squashes, cordials, spirits and other alcoholic drinks.

Fruit, Vegetables and Nuts
Tinned fruit, tinned vegetables, bananas, avocado pears,
peanuts, brazil nuts, hazelnuts, chestnuts.

Miscellaneous
Packaged, tinned and processed foods, semolina, stock cubes,
spreads and pastes.

Note. Alan also gave up smoking.

Allowed Foods

Fish
Cod, haddock, plaice.

Vegetables
Bean sprouts, beetroot, broccoli, cabbage, carrots,
cauliflower, celery, cress, cucumber, french beans, garlic, kale,
leeks, lettuce, mushrooms, onions, parsnips, peppers, peas,
potatoes, radishes, runner beans, spinach, spring greens,
spring onions, sprouts, tomatoes, turnips, watercress.

Fruit
Apples, apricots, blackberries, blackcurrants, cherries, goose-

berries, grapes, grapefruit, greengages, lemons, melon, oranges, peaches, pears, pineapple, plums, raspberries, satsumas, strawberries, tangerines.

Dried Fruit
Apples, apricots, currants, dates, figs, prunes, raisins, sultanas.

Fats, Oils
Flora margarine (contains milk solids) or other poly-unsaturated margarine, sunflower seed oil.

General
Heinz baked beans, maize meal, *Marmite*, brown rice, ground white rice, soya flour, *Protoveg*, split peas, split pea flour, tomato *purée*, lentils, butter beans, cornflour, home-made soups.

Nuts and Seeds
Almonds, walnuts, sunflower seeds, sesame seeds.

Herbs, Spices, Condiments and Flavourings
Mixed herbs (dried and fresh), oregano, fresh parsley, allspice, cumin, whole cloves, ginger, mixed spice, nutmeg, salt and sea salt, malt and wine vinegar, dried yeast, almond flavouring, *La Choy* soy sauce, vanilla flavouring, mustard, pepper.

Sweeteners
Fructose, date sweetener.

Drinks
Weak lemon tea, decaffeinated coffee, fresh or tinned unsweetened fruit juices, fresh or tinned vegetable juices, a rare glass of sherry or white wine.

Essential Supplements
Oil of evening primrose capsules six capsules (two, three times a day with meals). Vitamin B_{12} — *essential for non-meat eaters*. Multi-vitamin and mineral capsules are also important.

Recipes and Menus
This diet is quite taxing for a cook because it excludes the

basics for so many recipes – flour and all dairy produce. However, it is possible to overcome these initial difficulties. Rita Greer herself has written some excellent cook books, and she has also invented some very good substitutes for staple foods, e.g. pectin as a binder instead of eggs. She has even invented a Dundee fruit cake mix made without grains or eggs!

Rita Greer's products are available from various health food shops in the U.K., or direct from:

Cantassium Company,
225 Putney Bridge Road
LONDON SW15 2PY

These products include: rice flour, maize flour, carob powder, pectin, potato flour, fructose, salt-free baking powder. In addition, Rita Greer has developed various ingenious food mixes to save you the bother of concocting them yourself. She claims to have developed the first 100 per cent gluten-free bread mix. The other mixes include crumble topping mix, fruit cake mix, sweet biscuit mix, tomato soup mix, bran bread mix, pasta mix, instant bedtime drink, bolognese-style sauce mix, and a muesli base. All of these exclude gluten, saturated fat, refined sugar, and albumen (found in eggs).

Her recipes and menus are well set-out and beautifully illustrated in her various cook books. These are: *The First Clinical Ecology Cookbook; Fruit and Vegetables in Particular*; and *Rita Greer's Extraordinary Kitchen Notebook* (see *Further Reading*).

All the recipes in these books exclude gluten, cane sugar, cholesterol and are low in saturated fat.

Rita Greer, and many thousands of others, have tried and tested the recipes in these books and greeted them with enthusiasm. When Rita devised them, she made sure that they would appeal to the whole family, look good, smell good, taste nice, were nourishing, had enough fibre, were inexpensive, easy to make, and compared well with a food of a similar type.

It does take a while to get used to them, and some people might think their ingredients are a bit bizarre. However, with a bit of effort, they can be as appetizing as food made with more traditional ingredients.

Note. Rita's story is told graphically and amusingly in *A View On Diet* by Rita Greer (see *Further Reading*).

7 FOOD ALLERGIES

Both the Roger MacDougall Diet and Rita Greer Diet are
exclusion diets – they concentrate on leaving out certain foods.
Roger MacDougall's whole theory hinges on the belief that
M.S. people cannot tolerate foods containing gluten. Rita
Greer has gone beyond that and found that her husband Alan
was allergic to a great variety of foods, including seemingly
harmless ones like bananas, avocado pears, herring, shellfish,
and cashew nuts.

She has never suggested that other people with M.S. will be
allergic to the same foods as Alan. No two cases of M.S. are
exactly the same.

So, if you stick to either the Roger MacDougall diet or the
Rita Greer diet religiously, there is more than a chance that
you will be excluding foods that would be doing you no harm
whatsoever, and also eating foods that you are allergic to.

For example, it is not unusual for people to be allergic to
corn, tomatoes, coffee, and tea, to name just a few of the most
common ones. Wheat, and milk, are also commonly
responsible for allergic reactions.

There is a theory that the reaction to wheat is not because of
its gluten content, but because some Canadian wheat is
somehow faulty and can have an adverse effect on the body's

nervous system. If this were the case, there would be no good reason for not eating oats, barley and rye.

There seems no doubt that when the body's immune system has gone wrong, as in M.S., you can show abnormal reactions to foods which a normal healthy person could eat without any bad effects. Allergy symptoms include: tiredness after meals; palpitations; headache; nausea, bloating; high pulse rate; and sweating. In M.S. these can include cold legs; constricted breathing; difficulties with vision; lethargy; depression and a rapid onset of M.S. symptoms.

The offending food may give you a specific symptom. It may be, for example, that cane sugar always makes your eyes go hazy, or that grapefruit juice always makes your speech slurred. (These are my own reactions to cane sugar and grapefruit juice.)

There is only one sure way to find out which foods you are allergic to, and that is to test them, one by one. There are a miniscule number of allergy clinics where they can test your blood, or skin, but this is not practicable for most people, and anyway has no place in a self-help book.

To find out more about food allergies, read *Not All In The Mind* by Dr Richard Mackarness (Pan Books, 1976).

One of the most unwelcome truths about food allergies is that you are likely to be allergic to the foods which you crave most (for example, coffee, tea, sweet things, chocolate, cheese).

How to Test Yourself for Food Allergies

The principle behind testing for food allergies is that you can only find out which foods you are allergic to if you go on a cleansing fast first to clear out impurities from the body. Some doctors recommend a complete fast, but the one who formulated this one, Dr John Mansfield, reckons it is safe to start with a cleansing diet of lamb and pears, because practically no one is allergic to lamb and pears.

The Cleansing Fast: Lamb, Pears, and Spring Water
During the first *five* days you can eat only lamb, pears, bottled spring water, and sea salt – nothing else. You can eat them in any quantities and cooked any way you like, as long as nothing else is added. While you are casting off toxins into the

bloodstream, you will probably not feel very well. That will have passed by the fifth day. On the sixth day you should feel well enough to start testing the foods.

Note. This food allergy test contains many foods with saturated fat. You may feel it is worthwhile including them in the test to see what kind of reaction you do get to them. Cut the fat off the lamb during the first five days of lamb and pears only. If you are taking dietary supplements watch out for additives to them like sugar or yeast. Gelatin-covered capsules can be taken throughout the test.

Testing the Foods, One by One
This is not as arduous as it sounds. Once you have passed a food as safe, you can carry on eating it, together with your new food. For that reason you could be eating large and varied meals within a matter of days. There is no limit on quantity.

Day 1. Plaice, broccoli (fresh or frozen), turkey.
Day 2. Tomatoes, melon, beef.
Day 3. Tap water, rice, cod.
Day 4. Banana, soya beans, carrots.
Day 5. Milk, cabbage, chicken.
Day 6. Indian tea, apple, yeast tablets (Brewer's).
Day 7. Butter, leeks, pork.
Day 8. Potatoes, eggs.
Day 9. Wheat (as wholemeal bread). Two days are
and 10. needed for wheat as reactions to it are slow.
Day 11. Beet sugar (available in British Sugar Corporation packs), mushrooms.
Day 12. Percolated real coffee, grapes.
Day 13. Oranges, peanuts.
Day 14. Corn on the cob; glucose powder (made of corn). This again allows for a delayed reaction.
Day 16. Onion, lettuce.
Day 17. Cheddar cheese, spinach.
Day 18. Cane sugar, cashew nuts.
Day 19. White bread, coconut, garlic.
Day 20. Plain chocolate, grapefruit, dates.
Day 21. Courgettes or marrow, french beans, cauliflower.
Day 22. Oats, black pepper, rhubarb.
Day 23. Instant coffee, honey, asparagus.
Day 24. Tinned carrots, lemon, olive oil.

Day 25. Parsnips, avocado pears, natural yogurt.
Day 26. Rye bread, monosodium glutamate, prawns or shrimps.
Day 27. Saccharine tablets, cherries, brussels sprouts.
Day 28. Herring, almonds, raisins.

Some Guidelines on Food Testing

If you are testing three new foods in one day, separate each one by as many hours as you can manage. For example, test butter at breakfast time, leeks at lunch time, and pork at dinner time.

If you get no reaction, you can add that food to the next meal. For example, if you had tested lamb safely, and rice safely (Day 3), you could eat lamb, rice, and leeks on Day 7 for lunch. You would only be testing the leeks at that time, but if you got any reaction, you would know it must be the leeks.

If you *do* get a reaction, *you should not test the next food until you feel well again*, otherwise you could mess up the whole test. You might have to wait anything up to three days. If you do get a certain reaction, it is wise to re-test that food, but not for at least another five days, or more.

If you break the diet once, you might have to start all over again. It means sticking to each day's foods rigidly, and eating *nothing* else: no sauces, flavourings, etc.

You will notice that this list leaves out an awful lot of foods. It also leaves out cooking oils like sunflower seed oil. I think you risk nothing if you test, say sunflower seed oil and a polyunsaturated margarine very early on so you can use them for cooking.

This list does include all the most common foods which cause allergies. However, there is nothing to stop you adding more of your own if this list does not include foods you are suspicious about (like barley, hazelnuts, China tea?).

There is also no need to test other foods which fall within the same food 'family' as the ones on the list, e.g. brussels sprouts, as well as cabbage.

Isolating the Allergen

The important thing about this list is that it isolates individual ingredients. You may, for example, feel ill after eating a piece of cake – but what is it in the cake that is making you feel bad? It could be the cane sugar, or the white flour, or the butter, or indeed the cherries on the top.

With bread, you could find that you are allergic to the yeast, rather than the wheat. Be particularly careful about sugar. Beet sugar and cane sugar are not the same thing, and you could react differently to each.

Do not think that foods must be safe because they are 'natural'. It is possible for grapes, or apples, or almonds, or peanuts, for example, to give you an allergic reaction, even though they are not refined or processed or in any way adulterated.

Needless to say, this diet is very difficult to stick to, and is almost impossible socially. If you go out anywhere, it is safest to take a picnic of 'safe' foods with you, and explain the reason to your hostess. It is too risky eating out as you do not know what the well-meaning cook might have added in the way of sauces.

You must also avoid all alcoholic drinks, you must not smoke, and take no drugs whatsoever. It is also a sensible idea to let your G.P. know what you are doing, but do not be surprised if he takes it less than seriously. Most doctors are not convinced by the food allergy theory.

Once you have avoided a troublemaker food for several days, you will react much more strongly to it when you do eat it again. This is a good way of double-testing the suspect foods. Even though these foods give you a bad time, do not be surprised if you also long for them. The two together is a sure sign.

Avoiding Allergen Foods

This is the really hard part. By comparison, the month or more of food testing is easy. It is hard because the foods you are allergic to are most likely to be the foods you like best and eat most of. They are very likely to include some if not all the ingredients of cakes, biscuits and sweets. They may very well tally with the foods that the exclusion diets suggest you exclude anyway (wheat, cane sugar, milk, butter, cheese, real coffee – to name some of the commonest culprits!). On the other hand, you may discover a completely new list of foods that suit (or rather do not suit!) just you. On the other hand, you could find that you are not allergic to any foods at all.

8 WHICH DIET?

It may be very confusing having five separate diets all claiming to be good in the management of M.S., but in fact they share a lot of common ground.

Common Points Between the Diets
1. *Very little or no saturated fat.* The majority of the diets agree on no, or only very little dairy produce. What is included should be low-fat, e.g. skimmed milk, low-fat yogurt, low-fat cheese.
2. *Fish.* Unanimously applauded.
3. *Vegetables, legumes and pulses.* All very good. These should be fresh; raw wherever possible, or lightly cooked. Go for dark green leafy vegetables. Salads are highly recommended.
4. *Fruit.* Fresh, not tinned.
5. *Nuts, seeds and seed oils.* All very good (but watch out for peanuts). Should be unsaturated and untreated.
6. *No refined carbohydrates, refined sugar, processed or packaged foods.*
7. *No smoking.*

The Major Disagreements Between the Diets

1. *Gluten in grains: wheat, barley, oats, rye.* Roger MacDougall and Rita Greer say that these should be absolutely avoided. The others approve of whole grains. Try the food allergies test to find out if you are allergic to any of them.

2. *Lean meat; liver and other offals.* All but Rita Greer approve of these. As they provide a very rich source of arachidonic acid, vitamins, minerals and protein, only exclude these if you are certain that they make you feel bad. If not, they should be an important part of your diet.

3. *Sugars.* Some approve of raw honey and raw cane sugar. Rita Greer bans all cane sugar and honey. All of them ban refined sugar. Test yourself for raw honey; beet sugar, and cane sugar: it would be a pity to cut them all out unnecessarily.

4. *Alcohol.* Some allow it in moderation; others ban it completely. You may find you have an allergic reaction to certain drinks. Alcohol tends to inhibit the conversion process of the essential fatty acids, and to deplete the B vitamins in the body. It is better avoided.

So Which Diet?

The most important thing is to cut out saturated fat in dairy foods and fatty meats and replace it with unsaturated fat from vegetable oils. Probably the easiest diet is the essential fatty acid diet (see page 49) as it has been specially designed for people with M.S. and it is simple to stick to. If you remember to cut out all saturated fat, eat a lot of fish, liver, fresh fruit and vegetables, eat only natural wholefoods which are unrefined and unprocessed, and have a fresh raw salad a day, you will be eating a healthy balanced diet that is also doing you good.

9 VITAMINS, MINERALS AND M.S.

There are two main reasons why it is a good idea to take vitamin and mineral supplements. The first is that the diet you have been eating may have been deficient in vitamins and minerals. Diets containing a lot of refined and processed foods are most likely to be lacking.

The second, and more important reason, is that research has shown that various vitamins and minerals play a vital part in the various stages of the biochemical conversion process of the essential fatty acids. The four most important supplements for this function are:

1. Vitamin C.
2. Vitamin B6 (also known as pyridoxine).
3. Vitamin B3 (also known as niacin, nicotinamide, nicotinic acid).
4. Zinc.

These are substances, known as co-factors, which are involved in the manufacture of the end-products of essential fatty acid biochemistry – prostaglandins. (See section on prostaglandins and the biochemical conversion process page 25.)

These particular vitamins and minerals act as catalysts;

they make it possible for the various conversion stages to operate normally. Without these substances, the chemical reactions in the body are either slowed down, or sometimes stop altogether.

In addition, vitamin E is also vital, but for different reasons. This prevents the conversion of unsaturated fats to toxic materials. It is, therefore, an essential supplement if you are on a diet rich in essential fatty acids.

The above vitamins and minerals are the most important, but there is some research to show that other vitamins and minerals can have beneficial effects in diseases affecting the nerves and muscles.

The B-Group of Vitamins

B_6 and B_3 are essential for the biochemical conversion process of essential fatty acids; but the other B vitamins may be important too in M.S.

Vitamins B1 (Thiamine) and B2 (Riboflavin)
There is some research to show that polyneuritis occurs with B_1 deficiencies, and people with M.S. have been found to be low in B_2. B_1 is thought to be effective in improving conditions like neuritis, with numbness of the hands and tingling of the hands and feet. A B_2 deficiency can be connected with eye problems (e.g., retrobulbar neuritis, blurred vision), and to nervous symptoms like numbness, tremor, and the inability to pass urine.

Vitamin B3 (Niacin, Nicotinamide, Nicotinic Acid)
It is thought that people with M.S. are lacking in this vitamin. B_3 forms part of the body's enzyme systems and is essential for the biochemical conversion processes that go on in the body.

Vitamin B6 (Pyridoxine)
B_6 seems to play an important role in the health of muscles and nerves. It is necessary for the first stages of the bio-chemical conversion process of essential fatty acids.

Vitamin B12
Deficiencies in B_{12} can sometimes produce a disease which mimics M.S.: a shuffling gait or paralysis may occur, but are always associated with severe anaemia.

Pantothenic Acid
In certain laboratory animals, pantothenic acid deficiency has produced symptoms including the loss of the myelin sheath and degenerative changes in the spinal cord and peripheral nerves. The need for pantothenic acid is increased under stress, and is a good anti-stress supplement.

Choline and Inositol
Choline is concerned with the metabolism of fats. It helps in the production of lecithin (phospholipids). Inositol, too, aids in the metabolism of fats and seems to have some effect on muscular tissue. It has been found to correct some of the nerve disorders which can occur in diabetics.

Folic Acid
Folic acid appears to be concerned with helping new cells to form. It is very important in making blood and in keeping the intestines in good condition. Recent work has shown that it is also vital in maintaining healthy nerve function. Several studies have indicated that lack of folic acid is the commonest vitamin deficiency. It, therefore, should be taken as a supplement by people with M.S.

Biotin
Required by the body to assist in the metabolism of fats. Deficiency can cause a disturbed nervous system.

B-Vitamin Foods
You will notice that the foods rich in the B vitamins are all highly recommended in the Essential Fatty Acid Diet (see page 49). Liver, kidneys, other offal, yeast, wheatgerm, and dark green leafy vegetables are the major sources.

1. *Vitamin B1*: yeast; wheatgerm; unrefined cereals; bran; peas; beans; egg yolk; liver; kidneys; pork.
2. *Vitamin B2*: yeast; liver; leafy vegetables; heart; beef muscle; veal; chicken; apricots; tomato; milk.
3. *Vitamin B3*: liver; meat; fish; yeast; wheatgerm; eggs; nuts.
4. *Vitamin B6*: Yeast; liver; rice; peas; beans, lentils; peanuts; fish.
5. *Vitamin B12*: liver; kidneys; meat; fish; milk; cheese, eggs.

6. *Folic acid*: dark green leafy vegetables; liver; kidneys; beef; wheatgerm.
7. *Pantothenic acid*: yeast; liver; kidneys; wheatgerm; peas; soya beans; unrefined cereals.
8. *Choline and inositol*: wheatgerm; liver; brains; kidneys; heart; yeast; eggs; oatmeal; beans; peas; asparagus; brussels sprouts; cabbage; carrots; spinach; turnips; potatoes; grapefruit; oranges; peaches; peanuts; strawberries; soya lecithin.
9. *Biotin*: yeast; liver; kidneys; egg yolk; molasses; peas.

B-Vitamin Deprived Foods

The B vitamins are lost almost totally from wheat in the refining process. So white bread and white flour and all products made with white flour are deficient in the B vitamins. Wheatgerm is a major source of the B vitamins, so when this is discarded, so are the B vitamins. Other refined cereals suffer a similar fate.

All the B vitamins are water-soluble. They are not stored in the body and must be taken daily. These vitamins are vulnerable to heat, air, and water in cooking. If you cook foods in too much water, the B vitamins will get thrown away with the discarded water down the drain. A lot of B6 and folic acid is destroyed by heat in the cooking process, and some B vitamins get lost when the food is exposed to light.

Common Drugs

Alcohol, coffee and other drinks containing caffeine have a nasty way of depleting the body of the B vitamins. These stimulants appear to increase the loss of nearly all nutrients which dissolve in water. Research in the U.S.A. has shown that caffeine creates a shortage of inositol in the body.

Many of the B vitamins are also made by bacteria in the intestine, but if you are taking an antibiotic this will destroy the bacteria involved in this process.

The contraceptive pill depletes the body of B6.

B-Vitamin Supplements

The above facts should be enough to convince you that taking vitamin B supplements is to be recommended. The B vitamins are synergistic, which means that they work better when they are taken with each other. They probably also work better taken with other vitamins and minerals. Be particularly careful *not* to take B1 on its own.

All the B vitamins can be taken in capsule form by mouth, except B12 which doctors say often only works by injections. This is because a common cause of B12 deficiency is not a lack in the diet but a disease of the stomach, which means that the vitamin cannot be absorbed into the body from the gut.

B-Vitamin Doses

B1. An adequate amount for healthy people is thought to be 1mg a day. However, Adelle Davis, the American nutritionist, suggests 5mg a day for adults. Commercial tablets of the vitamin B complex include B1 at 2-5mg per tablet. At high doses, B1 is toxic. (Above 100mg or so a day.)

B2. An adequate amount is thought to be between 1.7mg and 5mg a day for adults. Commercial tablets do not usually exceed 5mg, but megadoses are available in tablets of up to 100mg each.

B3. Nutritional authorities consider that an intake of from 20mg to 30mg a day is needed by adults. Commercial tablets can contain doses of 7.5mg up to 166mg.

B6. An adequate amount for normal healthy people could be as little as 2-3mg daily, but people with M.S. should take much higher doses than this. Women on the contraceptive pill, or who suffer pre-menstrual tension, should take especially high doses. B6 is available commercially in doses up to 100mg per tablet. 200mg a day is safe.

B12. In Britain B12 is available on prescription as *Cytamen* in ampoules of 1mg. This can be injected once a week. Injections are only strictly necessary for people suffering from pernicious anaemia. By mouth, tablets can contain 5-10mcg.

Pantothenic Acid. The daily requirement is set at 10mg. Commercial tablets safely go up to 50mg per tablet.

Choline and Inositol. The requirement is uncertain but may be fairly high; 650mg daily for choline, 1000mg for inositol. Commercial tablets go up to 100mg per tablet. You could take up to 1000mg per day safely.

Folic Acid. 0.5mg daily is usually recommended, but anything up to 10mg a day is safe.

Biotin. The daily requirement is not known, but large amounts are synthesized within the body.

Vitamin C

Vitamin C is an essential dietary supplement. It is not stored in the body, but must be taken daily. It has two vital functions connected with M.S. Research has shown that it stimulates the formation of prostaglandins when taken with essential fatty acids, vitamin B6, and zinc. Vitamin C particularly helps the conversion process of dihomo-gamma-linolenic acid to prostaglandins. The second vital function of vitamin C is as an anti-oxidant in a diet rich in essential fatty acids.

Vitamin C is also well known as a detoxifying agent, and as a therapy for infections. It helps the body to defend itself against any foreign substance reaching the blood, and increases the bacteria-destroying ability of the white blood cells.

Foods Containing Vitamin C

The richest sources are rose hips, black and red currants, strawberries, and citrus fruits. However, the vitamin C content is destroyed by cooking, both by heat and the loss in the water thrown away after cooking.

Vitamin C Supplements

The minimum dose for an adult would be about 150mg daily, but people with M.S. should take far higher doses. This cannot be supplied just from food, so you should take a vitamin C supplement.

Dose

Vitamin C is non-toxic, and there is no risk in taking high doses. In Britain, the highest-dose tablets available are 1000mg (1 gram) per tablet. Taken twice daily, this dose is quite adequate.

Vitamin E

Vitamin E is essential to prevent oxidation of unsaturated fats to dangerous peroxides. It probably also reduces the conversion of essential fatty acids to toxic substances. So it is vital that you take enough vitamin E if you are eating a diet high in essential fatty acids and taking evening primrose oil capsules.

It is also important to take vitamin E supplements if you are on a gluten-free diet, as wheatgerm is the richest source of this vitamin.

Red blood cells break down when essential fats which form the cell structure are harmed by oxygen, due to a lack of vitamin E. Similarly, muscle cells can be destroyed without enough vitamin E. Muscular weakness can happen if they are not supplied with enough vitamin E, and the muscles can suffer from an increased content of calcium.

Foods Containing Vitamin E
Apart from wheatgerm, it is also found in the germ of other cereals, and in vegetable oils.

Vitamin E is largely lost in refined wheat and processed cereals, and when vegetable oils are hydrogenated, most of their vitamin E content is lost.

Vitamin E Supplements
If you have been eating refined and processed foods, there is a risk that your diet has been lacking in vitamin E. The minimum daily requirement is about 30mg. This vitamin is non-toxic and can be taken in high doses. It is efficiently stored in the body. It can be taken in doses of up to 600 i.u. (international units) per tablet, or 1,800 i.u. a day.

Vitamin F
This is an old name for the essential fatty acids, which is now beginning to come back into vogue (although vitamin F is not, strictly, a vitamin). The commercial capsules calling them-selves vitamin F are made of evening primrose oil (*F-500* and *Gamma*). These have almost exactly the same composition as *Naudicelle* and *Efamol G*.

Evening primrose oil capsules are the richest and easiest source of the essential fatty acids. They contain the unique and vital gamma-linolenic acid. (See Chapter 4 on Evening Primrose Oil.)

There are no foods which contain this, so it can only be taken as a dietary supplement. *Naudicelle* can be obtained from:

Bio-Oil Research Ltd.
Royal Oak Building
High Street
CREWE Cheshire CW2 7BL.
England (Tel: 0270-213094)

Efamol G can be obtained from:

Efamol Ltd.
40 Warton Road
LONDON E15 2JU
England
(Tel: 01-555 9042)

Lecithin

Lecithin plays a vital role in the metabolism of fats. In her book *Let's Get Well*, (see *Further Reading*) Adelle Davis says that autopsy studies on M.S. people showed a marked decrease in the lecithin content of the brain and myelin sheath covering the nerves, both of which are normally high in lecithin. The lecithin in people with M.S. is also, apparently, abnormal containing saturated instead of unsaturated fats.

Lecithin is continuously produced by the liver, passes into the intestine with bile, and is absorbed into the blood. It aids in the transportation of fats, helps the cells remove fats and cholesterol from the blood, and serves as a structural material for every cell in the body, particularly in the brain and nerves.

Lecithin consists of several substances which require essential fatty acids and choline and inositol for their structure, and numerous other nutrients to synthesize them. If these other raw materials are in short supply, lecithin is not manufactured efficiently in the body. These other nutrients include vitamin B6, and magnesium.

Lecithin Supplements
Lecithin supplements in capsules, tablets or granules can easily be added to the diet. Capsules of 200mg, six a day, are adequate.

Cod Liver Oil

Cod liver oil, in either capsule or liquid form, is an excellent supplement as it is a rich source of alpha-linolenic acid. This is particularly helpful if you do not eat much fish. It is also a very good source of vitamins A and D, which are also necessary.

MINERALS AND M.S.

Minerals are an essential part of a diet which is high in essential fatty acids. They help the biochemical conversion process in the body, and this complex vital function may not work efficiently without them.

Preliminary research has shown that zinc is essential for the synthesis of the essential fatty acids into prostaglandins. Copper, manganese, iron, magnesium and selenium may also have important roles to play.

Both the gross and the trace minerals are essential to man and the vast number of chemical reactions which are going on in the body all the time would not function properly without them.

Zinc

Zinc is a component of more than eighty body enzymes and hormones. It is essential for the first stages of conversion of essential fatty acids through to prostaglandins, and probably for a later stage as well.

Food Sources of Zinc

These tally with the foods rich in the B vitamins, and the foods recommended in the Essential Fatty Acid Diet: liver; kidneys; most meats; fish; shellfish; (oysters score highest); green leafy vegetables. Foods with almost *no* zinc content whatsoever are refined foods such as white sugar and white bread. The cheapest foods tend to be lowest in zinc. For that reason, people on low-income diets could be suffering from a zinc deficiency. There is some evidence too that people who have suffered physical injury or disease increase their excretion of zinc. Alcohol, corticosteroids and the contraceptive pill also cause the loss of zinc from the body.

Zinc Supplements

If you are eating enough of the foods rich in zinc, there may be no need to supplement your diet with zinc. However, since it is so necessary it would be safe to take tablets containing 2.5mg or 5mg of zinc. This is sold commercially as either zinc gluconate or zinc sulphate, either of which is fine.

Copper

One of the fundamental roles associated with the enzymes which contain copper is the protection of the body's cells from the damage caused by oxidizing agents. Lack of copper decreases the efficiency of detoxification, so that poisons can gradually build up in the body. Copper has a host of other functions, some connected with the body's use of iron.

Food Sources of Copper
Again, the richest sources are: fish; shellfish; (oysters and lobster have a very high content); liver; kidneys; heart; brain. Nuts, seeds, vegetables, raisins and prunes are very good sources too. (Poor sources of copper are: milk and dairy products; breakfast cereals; sugar; rice; refined flour.)
    If you are eating the source foods regularly, you should be getting enough copper and supplements should not be necessary.

Iron
The main function of iron is to do with carrying oxygen around the body. It is a constituent of haemoglobin, the red pigment of blood which carries oxygen. When iron is lacking, it means that less oxygen is carried to the cells. Oxygen deficiency makes you feel fatigued. Iron is also a constituent of some other essential enzymes in the body.

Foods Rich in Iron
The best sources are: meat and offal (kidneys and liver score high); vegetables; pulses (haricot beans and lentils high); and cereals, bread and flour (all unrefined). Iron is most easily assimilated from meats. The iron that is added to refined white bread is inadequate. The average Western diet provides from 10-15mg of iron per day, but only between 5 and 10 per cent of this is absorbed. Absorption is even less if meat is excluded. Iron supplements may therefore be necessary.

Magnesium
A deficiency of magnesium upsets the nerve-muscle functions and can be associated with tremor, convulsions, over-excitability and behavioural problems. A group of healthy volunteers who went on a diet deficient in magnesium developed muscle spasms and weakness, involuntary twitching and inability to control the bladder. These symptoms all went away when they took magnesium again. Some M.S. people in the U.S.A. reported that supplements of magnesium got rid of foot cramps.
    Magnesium is closely related to calcium and phosphorus in

its metabolic functions. Both calcium outside the cells and magnesium inside the cells are important in helping to transmit nerve impulses to muscles.

Food sources of Magnesium
Soybeans; dried Brewer's yeast; almonds; brazil nuts; wholewheat flour; peanuts; brown rice; dried figs. It is very low in white flour, white bread, milk, eggs, cheese and meat. A diet overbalanced towards refined carbohydrates and processed foods may well be deficient in magnesium.

Magnesium Supplements
If you have been eating a lot of refined and processed foods, it may be necessary to take magnesium supplements. Commercial tablets including magnesium contain doses of about 75-150mg.

Selenium

Selenium is one of the body's protectors. It is present in an enzyme called glutathione peroxidase (GTP). The various substances which attack cells are rapidly destroyed by GTP before they can cause any damage. Lack of selenium reduces the efficiency of GTP, and body cells are then open to danger. The white blood cells also contain high amounts of GTP. Selenium alone is probably not enough to protect the body; vitamin E is essential too. Like vitamin E, selenium is a powerful anti-oxidant.

Food Sources of Selenium
The best sources are the foods where the other trace minerals* are found; that is: offal (liver, kidneys, brain, heart, sweetbreads); seafoods; nuts; vegetables; fruit; unrefined cereals.
    Selenium is lost when food is refined and processed.

Manganese

Manganese is necessary for lipid metabolism, control of nervous irritability, and for proper bone growth and development. This mineral is directly associated with the defence mechanisms of the body. A fundamental function of manganese

* See *Further Reading* for books on minerals and health.

is in the synthesis of glycoproteins – combined sugars and proteins – in the body cells. These glycoproteins coat every cell, and protect them against invading viruses. Manganese is also necessary for the utilization of vitamin C.

Food Sources of Manganese
Wheat bran; most types of nuts; fresh green vegetables; alfalfa; tea. Manganese is lost in the over-refining of foods.

Orotic Acid (Also Known as Vitamin B13)
The vitamin-mineral bridge orotic acid is sometimes used in Europe in the treatment of M.S. It is used in the body in the metabolism of folic acid and B12, and is also vital for the replacement or restoration of some cells. It is said to play an important part in the body's utilization of minerals.

It is found naturally in such things as organically grown root vegetables, and whey, the liquid portion of soured or curdled milk. The Cantassium Company (in the UK) makes a range of B13 minerals: Calcium Orotate 500mg; Chromium Orotate 10mg; Copper Orotate 50mg; Iron Orotate 50mg; Magnesium Orotate 500mg; Manganese Orotate 50mg; Potassium Orotate 150mg; Zinc Orotate 100mg.

Commercial Vitamin and Mineral Supplements *
Some companies have come up with multivitamin and mineral tablets whose formulas are specifically designed for people with M.S. who are also on diets high in essential fatty acids.

RM Tablets
Roger MacDougall, who invented the Gluten-Free (Plus) Diet is involved with Regenics, a company which makes a tablet called *RM*, the contents of which are shown in Table 9.

Dose. Four tablets, three times a day with meals. In addition Roger MacDougall recommends Vitamin B12 tablets (10mcg), three times a day. *RM* tablets are obtainable from:

Regenics Ltd.
25-27 Oxford Street
LONDON W1R 1RF
(Tel: 01-437 7651)

* In U.K. only.

Table 4. Contents of *RM* Supplement Tablet

Nutrient	Content in mg
Choline bitartrate	10
Vitamin B1	2
Vitamin B2	1
Vitamin B6	6
Vitamin C	25
Vitamin E	7.5
Folic acid	0.015
Inositol	10
Nicotinamide (B3)	40
Pantothenic acid	12
Calcium gluconate	75
Magnesium carbonate	75
Lecithin	25

Cantamac

Table 5. Contents of *Cantamac* Supplement Tablet

Nutrient	Content in mg
Vitamin B1	4
Vitamin B2	2
Vitamin B3	166
Vitamin B6	10
Pantothenic acid	20
Vitamin E	30
Vitamin C	100
Calcium gluconate	150
Magnesium hydroxide	.150

These are made by:

Cantassium Company
225 Putney Bridge Road
LONDON SW15 2PY

(Available by mail order.)

'*Vital 4*'
The Cantassium Company also makes a product called 'Vital 4' which is specifically recommended to be taken with evening primrose oil capsules (which they market as *F-500*).

Table 6. Contents of *Vital 4* Supplement Tablet

Nutrient	Content in mg
Vitamin B6	50
Vitamin E	50
Vitamin C	250
Zinc gluconate	5

Efavite

Efavite is made by Efamol Ltd., who also make the evening primrose oil capsule *Efamol G*.

Efavite is designed to be taken with the evening primrose oil capsules, as they contain the essential 'co-factors' that help in the synthesis of the essential fatty acids. This tablet was not designed specifically for M.S., but for a variety of conditions where essential fatty acids are considered vitally important. However, it can well be used in M.S. Its contents are shown in Table 12 below.

Table 7. Contents of *Efavite* Supplement Tablet

Nutrient	Content in mg
Vitamin C	125
Vitamin B6	25
Vitamin B3 (niacin)	7.5
Zinc sulphate	2.5

Note. As *Efamol G* already contains 10mg vitamin E, this has not been added to *Efavite*. It can be obtained from:

Efamol Ltd.
40 Warton Road
Stratford
LONDON, E15 2JH
(Tel: 01-555 9042)

Some Conclusions

The disadvantage about the all-in-one multivitamin and mineral supplements is that some of the ingredients are in fairly low doses. On the other hand, you may prefer to choose the simplicity and ease of the all-in-one bottle. The all-in-one would also be cheaper.

However, if you do opt for a long row of bottles on your kitchen shelf, this is what it should include.

—— Vitamin C: up to 1g per tablet.
—— Vitamin E: up to 600 i.u.s per tablet.
—— Vitamins B1, B2, B3: choline, inositol, pantothenic acid, folic acid together. (See vitamin B 'Doses' page 80 for individual amounts. Beware of toxic doses.)
—— Vitamin B6: 10mg-100mg per tablet.
—— A multi-mineral tablet containing zinc, iron, copper, magnesium, selenium, calcium, potassium and manganese.
—— Cod liver oil: (vitamins A and D).
—— Lecithin: 200mg per tablet.

Plus   Evening primrose oil capsules (e.g. *Naudicelle* or *Efamol G*). Take two, three times a day, with meals.

Ideally, all the tablets should be taken at the same time, as they work best together.

Treatment with Colchicine, Evening Primrose Oil and Supplements

Work done by Dr David F. Horrobin in Canada has demonstrated that the drug colchicine has a beneficial effect when taken with evening primrose oil capsules and the supplements vitamin C, vitamin B6, and zinc. It has been found to increase the effectiveness of evening primrose oil two or three times in the biochemical conversion process from gamma-linolenic acid through to prostaglandins.

As a supplement for M.S. patients, it is prescribed in doses of 0.5mg per tablet, which is non-toxic and has none of the side-effects which can go with colchicine at higher doses. One tablet should be taken in the morning, the other in the evening.

However, colchicine is a drug and can only be prescribed by a doctor.

10   DRINKING AND SMOKING

Alcohol seems to have a bad effect on M.S. It inhibits the conversion process of the essential fatty acids, and nothing should be allowed to get in the way of this vital process.

Alcohol readily changes into saturated fat, and causes the amount of saturated fat in the blood to increase. It increases the need for vitamin B$_1$, pantothenic acid, and choline. Apart from that, alcohol can worsen M.S. symptoms, which can make you look like a drunk anyway. It can make co-ordination worse, and may affect standing, walking, finger movements, eye movements and speech.

It is possible too that you may have an allergic reaction to some ingredient in alcoholic drinks. Anyone on a gluten-free diet should not drink ale, beer and spirits. Sugar is added to many alcoholic drinks. Yeast can sometimes cause a reaction.

Far from being a stimulant, alcohol acts as a depressant. It could well make you feel low rather than high.

In some diets for M.S., alcohol is allowed in small quantities. If you find that a glass of good wine, or sherry does not make you feel bad, there is no harm in drinking these occasionally.

Alcohol is probably the most difficult thing to refuse

socially. Everyone expects everyone else to drink, and a glass of something is always being shoved into your hand at parties. However, if drink does make you feel ill, you must resist this kind of pressure. Insist on pure unsweetened fruit juices, or bottled water.

Cigarette Smoking

If you are going to go on a diet specifically designed for M.S., you must give up smoking. There is some evidence to show that cigarette smoking nullifies the good effects of a diet high in essential fatty acids. No one knows why this is so, but if you smoke and eat a diet high in essential fatty acids, you might as well not bother.

Smoking can also cause a temporary worsening of M.S. symptoms. One of the frequent effects of smoking is a lowering of skin temperature. This can aggravate M.S. where people tend to suffer from a feeling of cold in the hands and feet anyway. Also eye problems in M.S. can sometimes be associated with smoking.

The toxic substances from a single cigarette lower the blood vitamin C and destroy about 25mg of the vitamin.

Smoking can only do you harm. It is one of the greatest health hazards, and the most preventable cause of premature death. So, DON'T SMOKE.

11 CONSTIPATION

Constipation can be a problem in M.S., but if you stick to any of the recommended diets, you should not suffer from it because they are all rich in roughage (although a gluten-free diet does reduce the number of roughage foods available).

Foods rich in roughage include: onions; parsnips; celery; peas; beans; stringy vegetables, raw or lightly cooked; whole grains; wholemeal bread; bran; oatmeal; nuts; fresh and dried fruits.

Refined foods are low in roughage and will not help constipation.

Many people with M.S. have found that their constipation has been relieved after taking evening primrose oil capsules. The frequent use of oils like sunflower seed oil in cooking will help too. Also, drink a lot of water. Drink one glassful when you get up.

Dr Evers' tip for constipation is to chew whole fruit and take linseeds or soaked prunes before each meal. It is not a good idea to take laxatives as vitamins and minerals tend to get flushed out along with the rest.

12   FATIGUE

Fatigue in M.S. is not like normal fatigue which is caused by exertion. Fatigue in M.S. is not just tired muscles, it is the effect of the disease on the nerves which go to the muscles, and its effect on the sensory nerves.

The sensory nerves affect touch, sight, taste, smell and hearing. So, when you get fatigued, you can sometimes experience blurring of vision or slurring of speech.

Fatigue is brought on much faster in M.S. people than in healthy people, and it also takes much longer to recover from a bout of fatigue.

What happens when you get fatigued can differ from person to person. Fatigue often worsens existing symptoms, or can bring on symptoms that only happen when you are fatigued. On the other hand, old symptoms can come back, with the nasty habit of reminding you of your last attack. Severe fatigue can also bring on episodes of vertigo, or a flu-like feeling.

The Problems Caused by Fatigue

Fatigue is one of the most insidious symptoms of M.S., and one which has devastating effects in almost every area of life.

It may make it impossible for you to carry on working full-time; it makes it more difficult to bring up a family. Your partner may not understand why you always seem to be so 'lazy' or lethargic.

The roles which you had taken for granted, like mother, father, breadwinner, man-about-the-house, housewife, all have to be altered, and this can bring on some serious psychological and relationship problems, unless you and your partner learn how to adjust.

What Brings on Fatigue?

This can vary from person to person. It could be many things. You will probably be able to discover for yourself what makes you fatigued. Some of the most common things are exertion; eating a heavy meal; smoking; a hot day; a hot bath; humid weather.

Why Do You Feel Tired?

Any movement of any muscle requires energy. Energy starts from glucose, and to convert glucose into energy, the muscle needs oxygen.

Oxygen is brought to the muscle by the blood circulating through it. If there is not enough oxygen because of poor circulation, substances like lactic acid accumulate, and prevent the muscles from working. The oxygen supply to the muscles is increased when the blood-flow is improved by exercise.

Obviously, the whole process of energy production and muscle contraction is a highly complex one. However, it is important to understand the essential link between blood-flow, oxygen, and the working of the muscles.

Fatigue happens when the blood-flow, hence the oxygen-flow to the muscles, is inadequate.

How to Avoid Fatigue

Fatigue is not something you have got to continue to live with. You really can avoid it, but to do that needs will-power. Once you have found out what makes *you* fatigued, you can start planning your life accordingly.

Exercise

The first essential is to keep physically fit, and that means keeping the muscles exercised. This may sound surprising to you. Your doctor probably told you when you were first diagnosed not to do anything that over-tires you. True, you should never do any exercise to the point of exhaustion. However, if you do not do any exercise at all you will get fatigued much more easily than if you do.

Exercise tones up the whole system. After a session of gym, yoga or swimming, you should have more energy, not less.

You should be careful, though, not to overdo it. Your body will usually give you some early-warning signals when it is time to stop the exercise and rest. The ideal is to combine exercise with rest (see Chapter 13).

Rest

A rest some time during the day is highly desirable. This could be increased to twice a day during bad patches.

You do not necessarily have to go to sleep. Just lie down and relax completely. You could read a book, or listen to music, if you cannot go to sleep.

At other times, when you are just sitting down, you will feel more relaxed if you put your feet up.

The Rest-Exercise Programme

A specific rest-exercise programme has been formulated by the late W. Ritchie-Russell, a former professor of clinical neurology at Oxford University. You do not have to follow his programme to the letter if you prefer to devise a programme that suits your own particular needs. His therapy has had some good results. For full details read, *Multiple Sclerosis: Control of the Disease*, W. Ritchie-Russell (see *Further Reading*).

Sleep

It is common sense to tell you to get enough sleep. If you are going short on sleep, you are bound to feel fatigued. Try going to bed early. Tell yourself you will be in bed by a particular time every night, with perhaps one late night. This means being firm with other people. If you are invited out anywhere, politely insist on leaving when it is time for you to go. It will doubtless happen that your host or hostess will make you feel guilty about leaving so 'early', but guilt is better than fatigue.

If you can manage it, get some sleep during the day. An hour or so after lunch is usually the best time. Some symptoms of M.S. fatigue go away quite miraculously after a good sleep.

Heat

Heat is one of the main culprits of fatigue. Many, but not all,
M.S. people find that hot weather leaves them drained. Hot
baths have the same effect. Some people find that dry heat is
fine, but that humidity is intolerable.

The sensible solution is to keep out of the sun, and take
warm baths. It could also mean completely changing the kind
of holiday you and your family may have been used to. Your
need to be somewhere cooler and drier than where the rest of
your family wants to go to could cause problems, so you will
have to negotiate with them about where and when to go, and
find some kind of compromise.

Work

To change your job is one of the most difficult decisions when
you have M.S., but if your present job is strenuous and
stressful, you have to weigh up whether the price you will have
to pay in fatigue is worth it. If you carry on working full-time
in a demanding job, you may be too tired when you come
home to do anything else. The ideal is probably to find some
suitable part-time work, if possible, or change to a less-
demanding full-time job, even if that means stepping down the
career ladder a few rungs.

You do not have to give up work altogether just because you
have got M.S. It is likely to be pretty damaging to your self-
esteem and self-confidence if you do. Try and find the right
balance between work and the rest of your life.

Eating

A woman I know with M.S. gave me some invaluable advice
which works like magic in conquering fatigue: eat plenty and
often.

Being 'weak with hunger' has a particular relevance to M.S.
people. The symptoms of that unnatural fatigue (what some
people call 'feeling MSy'), creep over you when you begin to
feel hungry, and get worse as you get hungrier. If you go
without breakfast, you could be feeling deathly by mid-
morning.

Of all the things that bring on fatigue, this is the easiest to
overcome. If you are not at home with easy access to the larder
or fridge, it is no problem to keep a supply of emergency
rations with you all the time.

Be careful what foods you eat as snacks. Stodge (cakes, biscuits) are going to do you no good at all. Far better to assuage those pangs with things like raw carrots, a banana, dried or fresh fruit, or wholemeal toast (see Chapter 5 on diet).

Weight

After telling you to eat whenever you feel a first pang of hunger, it might seem odd to suggest that you lose weight. Yet, there is no need to be overweight if you eat just to satisfy hunger, and eat a balanced, healthy diet. If you are over-weight, you are likely to get fatigued more quickly, because of the excess bulk you are carrying.

Smoking

This habit can worsen M.S. symptoms (see Chapter 10).

Peace of Mind

M.S. fatigue can come on not just after physical exertion, but after mental exertion. When your brain gets tired, it feels a bit like a run-down car battery. So, it is just as important to rest your mind as to rest your body. One solution is to take up meditation, where you are taught how to empty and still the mind. Yoga would have the same effect.

Alternatively, you could make sure you spend time doing the things that relax your brain and still the mind. This could be a variety of things, like tending plants and flowers; in fact, any hobby that is creative and takes you out of yourself. Watching TV seems an effective way of relaxing the brain.

Help from Other People

Ask for help when you need it. It is better to do that than do a job yourself which leaves you drained. Other people are usually willing to help as long as you approach them the right way and you are not making constant demands on them.

Planning Your Life-style

All the remedies for fatigue in this chapter can only work if you plan your life-style carefully, negotiate these needs with other people around you, and you take a firm stand when it looks like you are going to be put in a position of doing some-thing you know brings on fatigue.

If you know that long car journeys, parties, or shopping expeditions make you exhausted, you will have to re-organize your life in such a way that you do not make long car journeys, you do not stay late at parties, or the supermarket delivers your groceries.

It means not accepting invitations three nights in a row; it means planning your day so you get enough time to exercise, and enough time to rest. It also means never skipping meals. However you need to organize your life with M.S., it will almost certainly be different from the life-style you led before.

13 EXERCISE

You may have been told by your doctor to take it easy and do nothing to tire yourself. In fact, M.S. can get worse if you are totally inactive. Of course, you should not do so much exercise that you get fatigued, but on the other hand, fatigue in M.S. can be due to not getting enough exercise. Your circulation gets sluggish, and oxygen does not get to the muscles (see previous Chapter 13). Everyone with M.S., no matter how disabled they are, can benefit from some kind of exercise.

Why Exercise is Important

—— It keeps muscles strong and strengthens weak ones.
—— It improves circulation and all bodily functions.
—— It keeps joints mobile and prevents stiffness.
—— It may help reduce spasticity.
—— It helps maintain maximum independence.
—— It helps prevent bed sores.
—— Generally, exercise gives you a feeling of well-being by toning up the whole system.

When you have M.S., it is important not to let the muscles fall into disuse. Once they have lost their tone through inactivity, it is hard to get it back again.

Apart from loss of muscle power, inactivity can also lead to depression, respiratory infections, blood clots, bowel and bladder disorders, pressure sores, and an imbalance in the body's chemistry.

What Exercise?

This depends on how badly disabled you are. Obviously, there are certain movements a recently-diagnosed M.S. person can do which would not be possible for a more severely disabled person.

If you are able to work and walk, there is no reason why you should not join just an ordinary gym or keep fit class in your local area. There are plenty of them, both run by the local education authority, and privately. If you do go to one of these, tell the instructor you have M.S. so you will not be forced to do things that are beyond your ability or stamina, and so that you can rest when you feel like it.

Any form of exercise will do you good. You do not have to go to a formal class. Swimming is the best form of exercise there is, and ideal for disabled people. One Australian woman I know with M.S. has built up her strength by swimming twenty lengths of her local pool every morning. She started by swimming just one length of the pool, and gradually built it up over the months. If the idea of going to a public swimming pool crowded with splashing children does not appeal to you, some local authorities have special swimming sessions for disabled people.

Any sport is good exercise, if you are still able to play them. Walking, too, is fine if you can manage it.

Special Gym Classes for M.S. People

Special gym classes for M.S. people are catching on all over the country. They were started in Burton-on-Trent by Joe Osborne of the Burton and South Derbyshire Independent Pool of M.S. Sufferers, and have been so successful, they have been copied elsewhere, by members of ARMS and CRACK. For full details of where these gym groups are, write to:

1. ARMS,
   71 Gray's Inn Road
   LONDON WC1X 8AR

2. CRACK
   M.S. Society
   286 Munster Road
   LONDON, SW6
   (Tel: 01-381 4022/5)

3. Joe Osborne
   Burton Independent Pool of M.S. Sufferers
   24 Beech Grove
   Newhall
   BURTON-ON-TRENT
   Staffordshire

If there is no gym group in your area, you could get together with some other members of ARMS and/or CRACK and start your own.

Going to a proper class is probably the best way of doing, or at least learning some exercises, as you have the discipline and sociability of a group. The groups are held on an average of once a week, although once a week is not really often enough to get real benefit. You should be doing some sort of exercise every day – even if it is only five or ten minutes. The once-a-week classes should be for longer sessions, however long you can manage without getting fatigued.

Exercising at Home
This does require a fair bit of will-power, but the results are worth it, and more severely disabled people who find it difficult to get out to group classes may only be able to exercise at home.

Many members of the Burton-on-Trent and South Derbyshire Independent Pool have kitted out their living rooms with bits of gym equipment, like wall bars, static bicycles, and rowing machines. (Some people feel virtuous just because they have bought a piece of gym equipment, but it will not do anything for you unless you *use* it!)

Burton-on-Trent Gym Class Exercises
Most exercises have to be demonstrated in person to be under-stood and done properly. These are a few which can be done correctly from a book. There are of course many more exercises than these, but you would need to be shown them by a trained instructor.

1. Lie on back. Draw up knees as far as possible. Give leg an extra pull by holding onto it with both hands. Try and press the top of your legs against your abdomen. Repeat four or more times.
2. Lie on back. Sit up. Touch your toes with your fingers. Repeat twice or more.
3. Lie on back, raise right leg as high as possible, then lower. Raise left leg, lower. Keep legs straight. Repeat twice or more.
4. Stand with feet wide apart, arms hanging loosely by your side. Do 'windmill' motions with both arms at the same time, brushing your ears and thighs as you go past them. Do four or more going forward, then four or more backwards.
5. Stand with feet wide apart, arms by your side. Bend to left, trying to get your left hand down past your knee. Then bend to the right, stretching down your right leg. Do not bend forward. Do four or more each side.

More Exercises to do at Home

The following exercises are a few taken from the book, *Multiple Sclerosis: Simple Exercises*, written by physiotherapist Gill Robinson specially for people with M.S. (See *Further Reading* for details.)

The ones included here are intended for people with M.S. who are still able to move unaided.

In Gill Robinson's book, there are other exercises included for more severely disabled people. As no two cases of M.S. are alike, it is not possible to give a set of exercises which would suit everyone with M.S.

1. Sit or stand. Take your arms out to the side and up above your head, and back down again (Figures 5, 6 and 7).
2. Lie down, sit or stand. With arms down by your side, reach as far down to your feet as possible, then back again, by leaning over sideways. Do each side in turn. Take care not to lean forward (Figures 8 and 9).
3. Lie down. Lift your head up as far as you can, then move your head down so that your chin is on your chest, then move it back again (Figures 10 and 11).
4. Lie down, face down. Raise each leg alternately off the

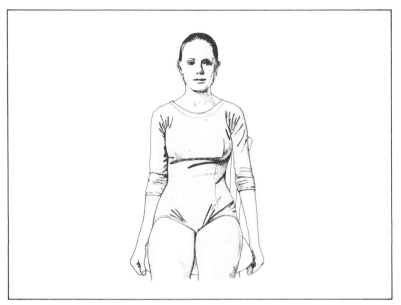

Figure 5.

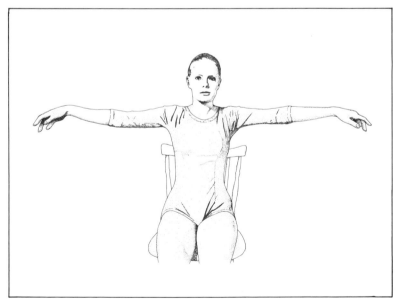

Figure 6.

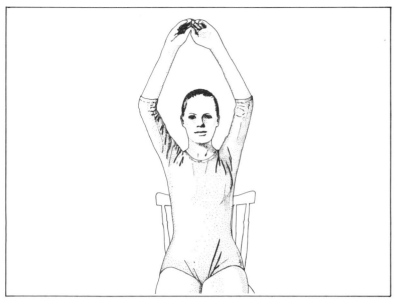

Figure 7.

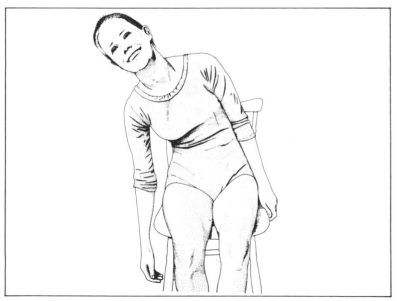

Figure 8.

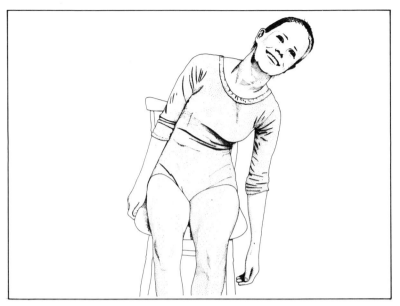

Figure 9.

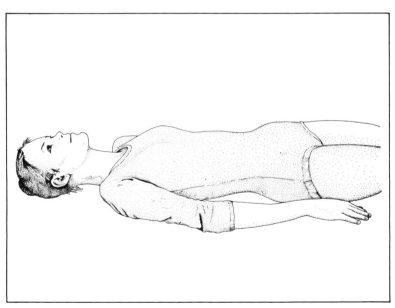

Figure 10.

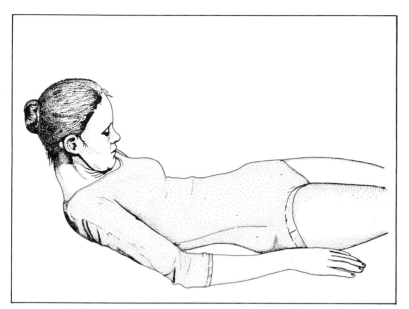

Figure 11.

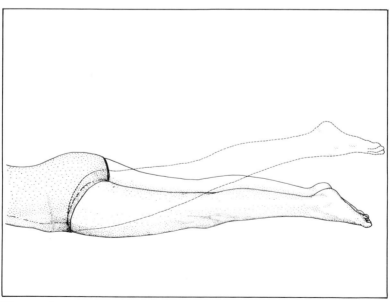

Figure 12.

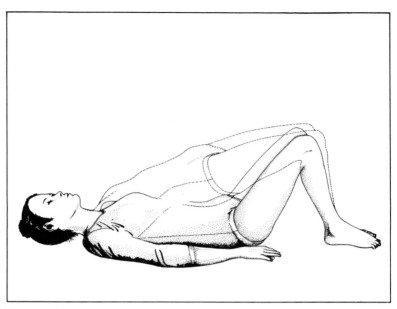

Figure 13.

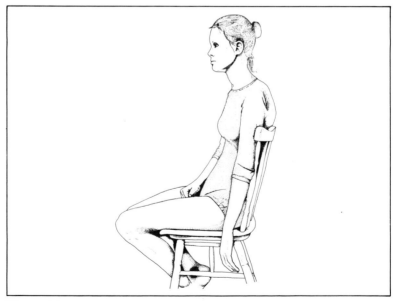

Figure 14.

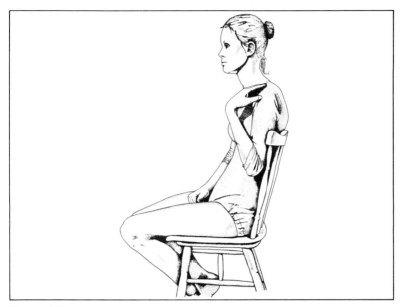

Figure 15.

floor, then down again. Then both legs together (Figure 12).

5. Lie down, knees bent, feet on the floor. Keep your feet and shoulders firmly placed on the floor. Raise your bottom into the air as far as possible (Figure 13).

6. Sit, stand, or lie down. Keeping your elbows as close to your body as you can, touch your shoulder with your fingertips and down again (Figures 14 and 15).

These exercises should be repeated up to ten times at first, gradually increasing this number as you become stronger.

Weights

If these exercises are very easy for you, you can make them more difficult by using weights. For some of the exercises you can use traditional dumbells. Alternatively, you can buy or make your own weighted bands which strap or fasten around the ankle. These are usually stuffed with lead shot.

A one-pound (450g) weight should make a difference. Weights have been used successfully in some cases to help control tremor or bad co-ordination.

The Powex Mark II Exercise Machine

People with M.S. who have lost the use of their legs may find it impossible to do any exercises involving the legs. However, a machine has been invented which makes it possible for people with paralysed legs to exercise them. You strap your feet onto the machine, and a motor makes the pedals go round on their own. The machine is driven by electricity, and plugs into an ordinary 13 amp socket, and is entirely under the control of the operator.

The Powex Mark II has an adjustable height; specially designed foot retainers; a variable speed; adjustable tension control so that the machine can be pedalled by the patient and adjusted according to progress; a hand control incorporating an emergency stop button. The machine is light to carry, and has a handle. It can also be easily stored.

It is available from the Burton and South Derbyshire Independent Pool for the sufferers of Multiple Sclerosis at:

24 Beech Grove Newhall
BURTON-ON-TRENT Staffordshire
(Tel: Burton-on-Trent 216638)

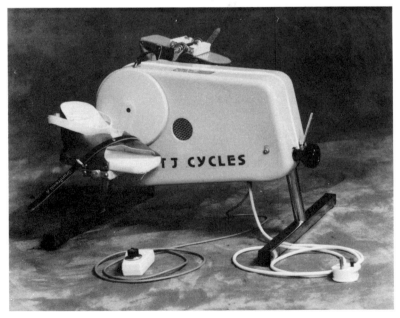

Figure 16. Powex Mark II Exercise Machine.

Physiotherapy

Physiotherapy does not strictly come under a self-help management plan. Even so, it is worth pointing out that physiotherapy has had some dramatically good results on some M.S. people.

If you have not yet done so, ask your doctor to refer you to a physiotherapist at a hospital with a good physiotherapy unit.

As well as giving you specific exercises to do at the hospital physiotherapy unit, they will probably give you a tailor-made exercise programme for you to do at home on your own.

As each patient would be given an exercise programme completely designed for their own needs, it is not possible to list a set of exercises here.

Many people with M.S. do not bother to see a physiotherapist. They may have decided that no one can do anything for them, and so have done nothing and seen nobody. It is simply not true that no one can do anything for you: physiotherapists are arguably the most helpful of all the things that are freely available to you on the N.H.S. (or you could see a private physiotherapist who would visit you in your own home).

As no two cases of M.S. are the same, it is not possible to list a set of exercises which a physiotherapist might recommend: it depends on so many individual factors. Some M.S. people have strong muscle tone with spastic movements, others have flaccid muscles with weak movements.

Physiotherapists always look at each patient individually to assess their own particular problem. When they have noted what is wrong and what is missing, they set about re-educating their patient to put things right and fill in what is not there.

You are taught how to stand properly, how to balance properly, how to walk properly, how to stand up from sitting and lying, how to position yourself to sleep, how to co-ordinate your movements better. Physiotherapists will also help you with things like being aware of your posture, your movements and your sensory perception.

There is a right way and a wrong way of doing all those things, and a physiotherapist will teach you the right way and stop you getting into bad habits. Their aim is to bring your body back into balance so you can move more normally and freely and enjoy an active life as long as possible.

One of the things that is *not* helpful is to increase the strength of the muscles that are strong already. This only makes the weaker ones weaker. If, for example, you are strong from the waist upwards, but weak from the waist downwards, there is the temptation to use your arms and trunk a lot, but not your legs and lower half.

There is a theory about 'associated reactions' which goes like this: the more you use your right hand, the weaker your left hand gets; the more you use your arms, the weaker your legs get. Take a look at yourself now and see which part of your body is over-compensating for another part.

When that happens, you should try and concentrate on the weak areas. The strong ones will look after themselves. That way, you have a chance of bringing your body back into balance. If you only build up the strong muscles, so that the weak ones stand no chance, the more out of balance you will be. That is why you should be careful not to put all your weight on your hands when you sit down or get up from an armchair. Use your legs as much as you can.

It is very important that if you have any disability at all you do see a physiotherapist as these things can really only be demonstrated in person. There is no doubt that the earlier you start physiotherapy the better. It will certainly prolong an active life.

Exercising Feet

Feet are often considered to be a vaguely amusing, not very important part of the body. Yet they are vital to the way you stand and move, and an important part of any exercise and physiotherapy programme for M.S.

There is an old Indian saying which goes 'You die from your feet upwards', and anyone who has experienced the icy blocks of M.S. feet will probably accept this.

Foot Reflexology

Reflexology is a rather complicated-sounding name for foot massage. The principle behind it is that each zone of your foot corresponds to a part of your body. This may sound unbelievable, but you can test it for yourself to see that it really does make sense. If, for example, there is something wrong with your stomach, you might be able to feel a sensation in your stomach while the stomach zone of your foot is being massaged.

Although it is possible for you or one of your family to learn how to do reflexology at a weekend course, it is probably better at first to go to a trained reflexologist. These are advertised in health journals etc. Some conventionally-trained physiotherapists are also beginning to use foot reflexology in their treatment of M.S. patients, with some very good results.

A reflexologist can tell what is wrong with you just by looking at and feeling your feet. By massaging particular areas, those corresponding areas in your body will be stimulated. A reflexologist working on someone with M.S. may well concentrate on the brain and the eyes, for example.

If you have numbness in the soles of your feet and toes, a reflexology massage can be pleasant. If, on the other hand, your feet are extra-sensitive, reflexology can be quite painful. This shows that the area is responding strongly. The pain will lessen, however, as you continue treatment.

Walk Barefoot
If your feet do feel like blocks of ice, or are numb, it will affect the rest of you and certainly affect your walking and posture. One way to stimulate your foot zones is to walk barefoot. Even better, walk barefoot on a coarse, grainy surface like coconut matting, every day. This is the next best thing to a reflexology massage.

Note. See *Further Reading* for books on reflexology.

The drawings in this chapter are reproduced from photographs which appear in *Multiple Sclerosis: Simple Exercises* by Gill Robinson (published jointly by ARMS and the MS Society of Great Britain and Northern Ireland — see *Further Reading*).

14 YOGA AND HEALTH

You may have thought that yoga was just a form of exercise where people get their bodies into peculiar positions. Yet, yoga is much more than just an exercise programme.

Hatha Yoga is based on the system of the relationship between the mind and the body. It concentrates on the whole person. As well as developing physical health, it also promotes mental health. It aims at getting the right balance between the mind and the body.

The word 'yoga' comes from the Sanskrit and means 'join or unite'. Hatha Yoga is about reaching a balance between the positive and negative poles within oneself. (*Ha* – sun – positive: *tha* – moon – negative.)

Disease

The yogic philosophy is that health is the natural state for human beings. Good health is when the body and mind are in a state of equilibrium. Illness, or dis-ease, is when the body and mind are out of balance.

There is a natural life force within all of us that is trying to do its best to keep us healthy. Yogis say that you do not become ill if you live a natural life. Even if you have been leading the unhealthy lifestyle of Western civilization, the body's healing powers are still there, just waiting to be given a fair chance.

Yoga and Multiple Sclerosis

Yoga has many advantages for someone with M.S.

—— Yoga may help the body's own self-healing mechanism and may slow down or even halt the disease process.

—— Yoga stills the mind.

—— Yoga increases energy and counteracts fatigue.

—— Yoga lifts the mood and counteracts depression.

—— Yoga has a good effect on the functioning of the endocrine glands, the circulatory and respiratory systems, and improves well-being.

—— Yoga does not need any special equipment and you can practise it daily at home.

The body's healing process works better when you are in a positive state of mind, and yoga helps you get into a positive state of mind. If your mind is at peace, your body can be used to the best of its ability.

The tension created by having M.S. can seize up the solar plexus (the network of nerves behind the stomach). This interferes with the movement of the diaphragm, and the body's energy flow is blocked. Yoga relaxes the body, opens up the diaphragm, and frees the energy flow.

Stress and tension may be both part of the cause, and the result, of having M.S. In many cases of M.S., something stressful is known to bring on an attack, or the first onset of the disease.

Stress, tension, and negative emotions are bad for your health and are likely to make you feel worse than you really are. It is vital to take up something like yoga to clear away the stress and switch your way of thinking from negative to positive.

If you are self-conscious about having M.S., you will be tense as a result. If you could only take your mind off a particular symptom or disability, you would probably be surprised how much the condition improved once you relaxed.

If you suffer from spasms, or spasticity, or clumsiness, for example, just think for a moment how those symptoms lessen when you are completely relaxed. Do not think about it too hard, though, because once you get self-conscious about it again, the tension will increase and so will the symptoms.

Negative Feelings
Negative feelings are known to undermine the health, lower the body's resistance to infection, and delay the healing process.

You know from your own experience how the emotions can affect your body. Winning the pools makes you feel on top of the world. Whereas bad news makes you feel ill, with perhaps symptoms of sickness, palpitations, a dry mouth, weakness, and so on.

Rage, fear, grief, sorrow, fright, jealousy, despondency or pessimism make you feel physically bad. Of these, fear is supposed to be the most noxious.

Conversely, the positive emotions such as love, joy, and compassion make you feel physically good.

The Negative Personality
This is the kind of person who is lacking in self-confidence and is full of self-doubt. They have no faith in their own powers, so they always go to other people for help. They are afraid of everything. They tend to fail, and they tend to see the worst in everything and everybody. They are selfish. They do not understand themselves or other people. They are morose, despondent, and peevish. They are always complaining about everything. They are the kind of people who say 'I can't'.

Most people can recognize at least some of themselves, at least some of the time, in this portrait. A person like this not only finds it hard to be happy, he is also likely to be unwell. However, the practise of yoga can transform the mind to thinking positively, which at the same time will have a positive effect on the body.

Yoga Exercises for M.S.
Any book on yoga will show you that there is a vast range of yoga exercises (asanas). None of them are harmful to people with M.S. How far these can be practised depends on the individual and the degree of disability.

People with M.S. often find it difficult to do a particular movement and hold a position – when they first start yoga.

With practice, however, many people with M.S. find they can make dramatic progress and find quite quickly that they can do some exercises they never thought possible.

Select exercises which fit in with your own condition. If you are a beginner, the best thing is to go to a proper class and be taught by a trained instructor. It is not really satisfactory to learn yoga just from a book, though well-illustrated books can be an aid to going to a class as well.

There are some classes specifically for M.S. people run by the Yoga for Health Foundation. Write to them at their head-quarters to find out if there is a group in your area. They also run residential yoga 'holidays' (weekends, weeks, or even months) at their H.Q. in the country, which is a beautiful old country house.

Yoga for Health Foundation
Ickwell Bury
Nr BIGGLESWADE
Bedfordshire
(Tel: Northill 271)

If you are still at the working/walking stage, there is no reason why you should not go to an ordinary yoga class in your area. Again, the Yoga for Health Foundation run many classes all over the country which are for anybody (who is a member). Local adult education centres often run yoga classes, or private teachers sometimes advertise their classes in the local paper.

If you do go to a 'normal' class, tell the instructor you have M.S., as there may be some exercises to begin with that you find particularly hard, such as those which require balancing on one leg. Do not cop out of doing these exercises; they are probably the ones you need to do most! The instructor will probably give you some extra attention on the exercises you find hard, so that you gain confidence and your ability to do them increases.

Yoga asanas tone up the neuro-muscular system of the body and keep it in full working order; they develop and control the respiratory system, increasing oxygen flow and vitality. The internal organs work better; the spine is kept strong and supple.

Yoga Exercises to do at Home

Once you are familiar with the basics of yoga, there are many exercises you can do on your own at home.

How to Relax

Relaxation is one of the most important things yoga can teach you.

Lie on a mat or carpet in a warm, draught-free room. Your legs should be at least one foot apart, with no tension in the ankles. The toes should fall outwards. Make sure your trunk is lying as firmly as possible against the floor, and that your arms are away from your sides, with the palms upwards.

Keep your head in a straight line with your body. If you feel uncomfortable, put a very small pillow behind your neck to take the weight, but make sure your shoulders are resting firmly against the ground.

Once in this position, think yourself through the whole of your body, telling yourself to relax each part. Pay special attention to the muscles of the face, especially the jaw, and around the mouth and eyes. If your teeth touch, you are not relaxed.

When you breathe, your abdomen should rise naturally as you breathe in, and fall as you breathe out. Never push the tummy out – let the rise be natural. However, you can pull the tummy muscles in gently on the exhalation. This movement makes sure the diaphragm is moving up and down. Practise for between five and fifteen minutes daily.

Some Simple Exercises

1. Lie on the floor, legs together, hands by the side, palms down. Breathing in slowly and deeply, bring the hands up over the head until they touch the ground (or as near as they can get to it). Breathe out slowly, retaining the position. Breathe in again, and slowly bring up the legs, bent or straight (preferably straight) as high as you can without straining. As you breathe out, bring down the arms. Breathe in again, keeping the legs in the air. Then, as you breathe out, slowly bring your legs down. Repeat two or three times.

In the illustration (Figure 17) Rachael Lack is using her stronger left leg to help the weaker right one.

2. Lie with your back to the floor. Bring your heels into your

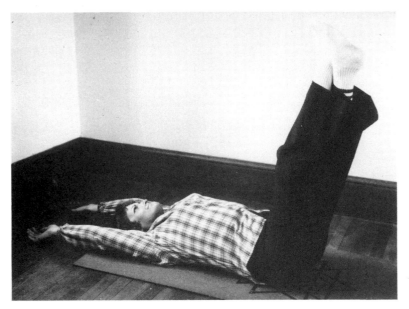

Figure 17. Yoga exercise 1.

bottom. Breathing *out*, bring your bottom – not the back – off the ground, by tilting up the pelvis. This means hardening the thigh muscles and the lower abdominal muscles. Then, breathing *in*, slowly drop the bottom and arch the back, so you end up resting on your shoulders and bottom. This is a very powerful movement which helps the spine and the hip and leg muscles. Repeat a number of times (Figure 18).

3. Go on to all fours, looking ahead. As you breathe in, drop the back and raise the head. As you breathe out, arch the back up and drop the head between the arms. Continue this a number of times. Then sink back on to your heels, bring your hands round by your feet, palms upward, and then let your whole trunk go forward so that your forehead is resting lightly on the ground. Stay in this position for some minutes, breathing gently (Figure 19).

4. Lying on your back, spread-eagle your arms to either side. Start with your legs together. As you breathe in, bring up one leg. Then, breathing out, swing it across your body onto the ground the other side (or as near to the ground as it will go). Turn your head in the opposite direction and keep your

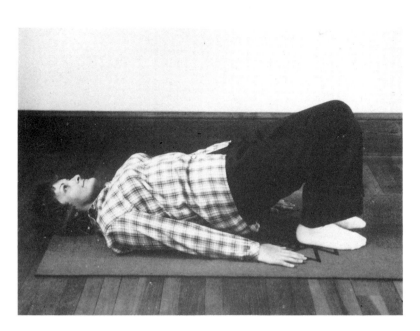

Figure 18. Yoga exercise 2.

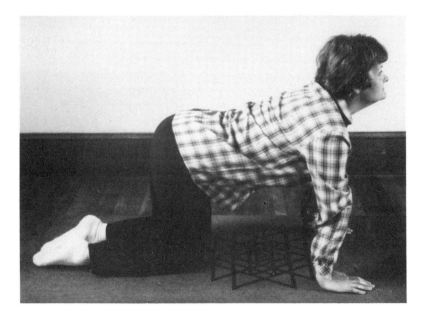

Figure 19. Yoga exercise 3.

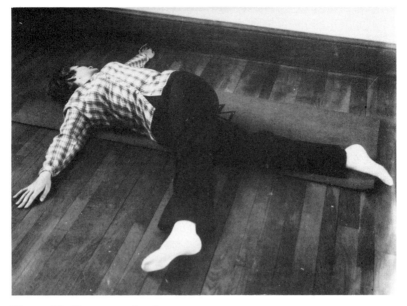

Figure 20. Yoga exercise 4.

shoulders on the ground. Hold this position, breathing normally.

Each time you breathe out, feel the leg coming nearer to the ground, or resting more heavily on it, the spine twisting a little bit more and the shoulders firmer against the ground. Breathe in, bring the leg up and back to the ground next to the other one, breathing out. Repeat with the other leg (Figure 20).

Some Points about Yoga Exercises

Do them slowly and thoughtfully. Visualize the whole process first. Tell yourself what you want to do and how you are going to do it. Keep your mind on the part of the body you are exercising.

Controlled inhalation and exhalation will help you do the movements.

Yoga positions are achieved through controlled relaxation. Some muscular tension is required to achieve the movements, but this is kept to a minimum, and you never need to strain or pull harshly.

Hatha Yoga has the opposite effect of many physical exercises. It does not tire you; on the contrary, you may find that, even if you are tired before you start doing the postures, you have much more energy afterwards. Fatigue should not be a problem.

You can take a rest whenever you feel like it during the exercises. Breathe very deeply from the abdomen. Finish each session with a fairly long fifteen-minute relaxation session. You should be completely refreshed after this.

Try and do some yoga every day. That way, you will keep up your positive mental outlook and physical condition. If you can get into the habit of ten minutes to half an hour first thing in the morning, it will set you up well for the rest of the day. Alternatively, half an hour's yoga at about 6p.m. will revitalize you after the day's work.

Breathe!

Correct breathing is one of the most important aspects of yoga. You may think that breathing is something that everyone does naturally. In fact 99 per cent of the population breathe incorrectly, with correspondingly ill effects on their bodies.

Breathing is the most important biological function of the body. Every other activity of the body is closely connected with breathing. To realize just how important breathing is, remember that you could live for weeks without food, days without water, but only a few minutes without air. Breathing is of primary importance to one's state of health, emotional outlook, and length of life.

Most people in the West take short, rapid, shallow breaths, but it is the deep, rhythmic breathing which brings health and energy.

Any shock makes people seize up. Notice how you breathe out with a sigh of relief when some ordeal is over. When people are tense, they tend not to breathe out enough. 'I held my breath' is a common phrase for being excited or nervous about something. Yet, if you hold your breath often enough, it is obvious that your body is not going to get the oxygen it needs for energy.

If the energy is not flowing properly, it will affect both your body and brain. You will get fatigued easily, feel run down and depressed. If you are breathing deeply and rhythmically, you will find it hard to be tense at the same time.

If you can learn how to breathe properly, this is one of the simplest yet one of the most important things in the self-help programme for the management of M.S. The first thing to learn is that you should breathe out through the nose, *not* the mouth. Also, shift your breathing from shallow breaths which use only the upper part of the chest, to deep, abdominal breathing. When you are doing it correctly, if you put your hand on your tummy you can feel it rise like a balloon, and then go very flat, without any effort.

When breathing deeply, you use the diaphragm. The diaphragm is the very strong muscle which stretches below the rib cage, separating the lungs from the internal organs.

If the breathing is corrected, and is co-ordinated with your movements, all your movements should become more normal.

M.S. as a disease demonstrates the total imbalance of body energy. It is within your power to redress some of that imbalance, and by breathing properly and co-ordinating your breath with your movements, you will be helping to correct that imbalance.

Once you have learned how to breathe properly, you can learn how to concentrate single-mindedly on the breath. This is a very effective technique for meditation. It stills the mind, clearing it of worries and anxieties.

You will probably need to go to a trained instructor to learn correct yogic breathing, meditating on the breath, and some very beneficial breathing exercises to help tone up the nervous system.

Pain

Pain is not a symptom that is commonly associated with M.S., yet about 13 per cent of people with M.S. do suffer from pain of varying severity.

This is one of the things your doctor should be able to help you with. There are pain-alleviating drugs which your doctor can prescribe for you, and you should consult him about these.

In Britain, there are now a hundred or so pain clinics at various hospitals and, if necessary, your doctor could refer you to one of them.

Much of the pain in M.S. is due to muscle spasms. You may find that doing yoga, or some other relaxation technique will help reduce the spasms and therefore lessen the pain.

15 POSTURE

Incorrect posture can only make your M.S. worse. It throws the body out of balance, and will have a bad effect on breathing, and the function of the internal organs. Below are a few hints on correct posture.

Lying Down
It is vital that you do not stay in the same position for a long time. You need to move or be moved every few hours to prevent bed sores, and keep your circulation going.

Lying on your back for long periods encourages spasticity. Lying on alternate sides will help prevent these problems.

Sitting Down
Sit on a chair where your feet can be flat on the ground. Your thighs should be well supported, and your ankles, hips and knees at right angles. Ideally, the chair should be deep enough so that your thighs are fully supported when your bottom is placed well back into the chair. This avoids pressure on the back of the knees.

The arm rests should be at a height where your shoulders are completely relaxed when the forearms are supported. The back of the chair should be high enough for your head to be supported when necessary.

To sit properly, your bottom should be well back into the base of the chair, and your back should be in contact with the chair back. Heels should be down on the floor, knees slightly apart, thighs well supported. Your shoulders should be relaxed, elbows slightly away from your body; forearms and hands well supported by the arm rests. Your head should rest comfortably on the back of the chair.

Standing Up from a Sitting Position

The difficulties many M.S. people experience can be lessened by following a few simple rules.

1. Any walking aid should be at hand, ready for use.
2. Wear shoes.
3. Make sure you are on a non-slip surface.
4. Put your feet slightly apart, flat on the floor. Pull them back towards the seat.
5. Place both hands on the chair arms and ease yourself so that your bottom is fairly close to the front of the chair.
6. Lean slightly forward, lifting your head and looking straight in front.
7. Push with both hands on the chair arms.
8. Push your heels down, straighten your knees and hips. Try not to put too much pressure on your arms and hands. You should use your legs as much as possible, otherwise your arms and hands will be disproportionately strong to your legs. Try and use your leg muscles as much as possible too when sitting down from a standing position.

Sitting Down from a Standing Position

Approach the chair. Turn round so you can feel the chair with the back of your legs. Feel for the chair arms with both hands. Slowly lower yourself down into the chair.

Walking

Try to keep a correct balance, though this is pretty hard when your body has been thrown out of true. It will be easier if you try and stick to some guidelines.

1. Your feet should touch the ground with the *heel* first, not the ball of the foot.

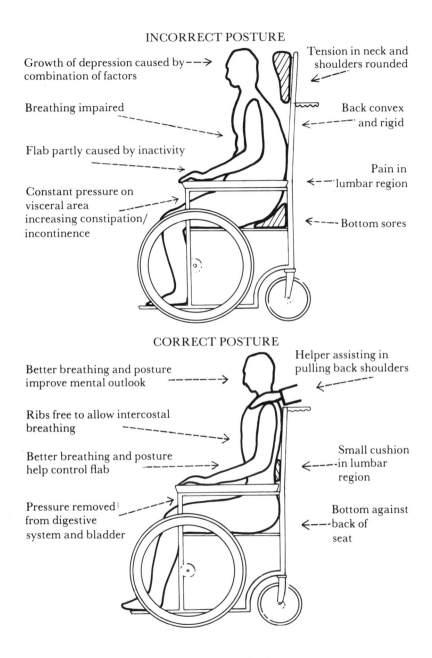

INCORRECT POSTURE

Growth of depression caused by --→ combination of factors

Tension in neck and shoulders rounded ←---

Breathing impaired

Back convex ←----- and rigid

Flab partly caused by inactivity

Pain in ←--- lumbar region

Constant pressure on visceral area increasing constipation/ incontinence

Bottom sores ←----

CORRECT POSTURE

Better breathing and posture improve mental outlook --→

Helper assisting in pulling back shoulders ←-----

Ribs free to allow intercostal breathing

Better breathing and posture help control flab

Small cushion ←----in lumbar region

Pressure removed from digestive system and bladder

Bottom against ←---back of seat

Figure 21. Good and bad posture in a wheelchair.

2. Direct your feet forwards. Make sure they are not splayed outwards or inwards.
3. Remember to breathe. The sequence should be *in* as the leg comes *up*, and *out* as the leg goes *down*.
4. Do not be self-conscious – relax. A lot of awkwardness and clumsiness in M.S. people is because they are self-conscious of their appearance and movement.
5. Look straight ahead, not down.

If you have a helper or a stick, try not to lean lopsidedly towards the aid. Once your body is thrown out of balance, it will try and compensate, and get even further out of balance.

Posture in a Wheelchair
Sitting in the wrong position in a wheelchair can make you feel worse. If you sleep in a wheelchair, it can make you feel depressed, impair your breathing, and make for flabby muscles, constipation, incontinence, tension in the head and neck, back pain, and sores on your bottom.

If you constantly slump in a wheelchair, you will be saddled not just with M.S. but with a host of other complications which need have nothing to do with the disease.

For the correct way to sit in a wheelchair, see Figure 21. It is not necessary to sit like this all day, although the position will get increasingly more comfortable. Sit like this for as long as you can, where possible with a helper to correct your position.

Sit right back in the chair, with your bottom against the back of the seat. Put a small, reasonably stiff cushion, about five inches deep, across the lower back. Tie it to the back of the chair with tapes. This enables the spine to be held in the correct concave shape, and the rib cage and chest are raised, which helps keep the breathing right.

16   PRESSURE SORES

Pressure sores are probably the most preventable condition connected with M.S. If you know how to avoid them, you need never get them. But once you have got them, they can take months to heal.

Pressure sores happen when you put constant pressure on the same spot for a long time. This constant pressure causes lack of circulation, and this lack of circulation means there is no oxygen or glucose getting to the area.

The most vulnerable places to get pressure sores are the buttocks and tops of the thighs, particularly if you are in a wheelchair. If you are lying immobile in bed, pressure sores can happen at any point where the body comes into constant contact with the bed, bed clothes or other parts of the body. These areas include the lower back, the shoulder blades, the insides of knees, hips, elbows, ankles, heels, toes, wrists, even ears.

The Warning Signs
The beginnings of a pressure sore can look as innocent as a bruise, or just like a small red patch. It may look like a blister or weal, and the skin may be broken open to expose a hole.

Whatever the sign, the pressure sore will feel painful and sore.

What to Do If You Get a Pressure Sore

Seek medical help IMMEDIATELY. It is not a bruise or a blister, and will get worse unless you get treatment for it.

Treatment

The usual person to treat pressure sores is a nurse, either in hospital, or the district nurse who will visit you in your own home. Although it is possible for you to buy the medicaments from a chemist and put them on yourself if you are able to.

The usual treatment is an antiseptic cream, such as *Conotrane*, rubbed gently into the skin surrounding the sore. This gentle rubbing is to get the circulation going. An antibiotic powder such as *Cicatrin* may be sprinkled on the skin. This has the effect of drying it and preventing the sore from becoming pussy. During the day, a pressure sore is usually left exposed to the air. But at night it is covered with a sterile dressing such as *Melolin*.

It is important to keep the skin clean and dry. Some people find a gentle rub with soap and water around the sore, followed by meticulous drying, helpful. But take care not to let the skin get too dry because infections can start in the cracks. If you do have dry skin it is better to use zinc and castor oil cream instead of soap, and to wash less frequently.

Various creams, ointments, sprays and powders are on the market to treat pressure sores, most of them only on prescription. But some people have found some home-made remedies work well, such as honey, honey and lemon, cod liver oil, or Friars Balsam mixed with zinc and castor oil cream. The paste is put on to the skin and left there, rather than rubbed in. Ultra violet light, and oxygen are also good remedies.

Things to Sit and Lie On

As well as medicaments to apply to the skin surrounding the sore, there are various mattresses, cushions, pads, etc. which are specially designed for immobile people. These work by relieving the pressure on one area by subtly helping you shift your position and thereby aiding the circulation. Their texture also prevents you from chafing your skin.

The most helpful aids are sheepskin, either as a wheelchair

or bed cover; ripple cushions and ripple mattresses; foam rings; gel cushions; air cushions; Sorbo pads; and water beds.

If bedclothes have caused soreness, you may have to use a cradle or sandbags to take them off the body. Nightdresses and pyjamas can cause soreness too. Ideally, you should be naked from the bottom down, as this is the most vulnerable area. Avoid hard metal bed pans; choose soft rubber or plastic ones instead.

Move, Or Be Moved, Frequently

The key to preventing pressure sores is to move, or be moved, at least every two to three hours. During the day, stand up frequently and, if you can, walk about. If you cannot stand on your own, ask someone to help you.

If you are bedridden, or immobile, ask someone to move your position during the night. This might sound like a chore, but it is less troublesome than coping with nasty pressure sores.

A healthy diet with lots of protein will also help prevent pressure sores (see Chapter 5).

17 INCONTINENCE

A fairly common symptom of M.S. can be weakened control of the bladder, due to the damage to the nerve pathways in the lower part of the spine. You may feel an urgent need to go to the toilet, frequently, even though there is not, in fact, much urine in the bladder.

Alternatively, some people suffer from bladder retention, when they cannot pass water, no matter how hard they try or how much they feel they want to. In more advanced cases of M.S., double incontinence (faecal incontinence) can sometimes happen too.

These are particularly distressing symptoms because they are surrounded in our society by feelings of embarrassment and shame. Some people I know with M.S. find the possibility of wetting oneself in a public place, not being able to find a toilet in time, or emitting an unpleasant odour, a worse handicap than, say, walking with a limp.

With the help of drugs, special pants and pads and other aids, it is possible to manage the problem of incontinence in such a way as to lead a near normal life. There are some things that work, and others which do not. This chapter lists some of the best – and worst-products.

It is worth pointing out that some people who were incontinent (e.g. Alan Greer) stopped being so after finding a diet that had a regenerative effect on them. You may find if you stick to the management regime suggested in this book, your symptoms of incontinence might improve.

See Your Doctor

Incontinence is one of the things your doctor can help you with. There are certain drugs available which can help a lot. There is, for example, one which does work in reducing the feeling of extreme urgency and will give you longer to get to the lavatory. Also, if you need a catheter, medical help is essential.

Your doctor should be able to help you with advice on other aids and equipment. If you do not have a social worker, the Social Services should be able to provide one for you (in Britain). Social Services departments, however, are not always as helpful and efficient as they could be. You may find that the aids and equipment they are prepared to give you are not as good as those available privately. A list of private suppliers is, therefore, included in this chapter.

Drinking

You may think that if you cut down on your fluid intake, your need to rush to the loo will be reduced. Not so. The trouble with drinking very little is that the urine becomes concentrated and smelly, which can be just as uncomfortable in a different way as a full bladder. You should drink at least five glasses of fluid a day – more (eight to ten) if possible. Drink more, earlier in the day. Do not drink anything for a couple of hours before going to bed. That way, you are less likely to be wet at night. If you wear a catheter, it is very important to drink a lot of fluid, otherwise it collects debris. A high fluid intake will wash away the debris.

Drinking an adequate amount is also essential to avoid constipation.

Coffee and Wine

Both coffee and red wine can irritate the bladder lining and make you feel more of an urge to pass water than you would otherwise. Other alcoholic drinks could have the same effect too. Coffee and wine are bad things in a diet for M.S. anyway.

Constipation

Constipation makes incontinence worse. The pelvic congestion caused by constipation presses on the bladder. So it is very important to avoid constipation. Drink a lot. Try a hot drink (water with lemon is a good one) first thing in the morning. Eat bran, fresh fruit and fresh vegetables.

Going to the Toilet

Make sure you empty your bladder completely. Stay there long enough to make sure there is nothing left. Women should lean forward to help empty the bladder thoroughly. It is also common sense to organize your life so you are not far away from a toilet. Before setting out on a journey or going to somewhere you have never been before, it is a wise precaution to find out where the toilets are.

Pads and Pants for Women

Women are at a disadvantage compared to men because there is no practical alternative to wearing pads and special pants. This can be a particularly demoralizing experience because you can feel as if you are regressing to babyhood. To avoid these feelings it is a good idea to choose pants which are as attractive as possible, and pads which are not ugly and bulky. With the right kind of pads and pants, you should be able to wear normal, fashionable clothes and keep your incontinence a private matter.

The urology unit at St George's Hospital in Tooting, South London has been testing a variety of pads and pants, and has found some to be good, and others to be bad.

Recommended Pants

The most important thing is to find pants which fit very well, otherwise there is a risk of leakage down the leg.

Kanga Pants fit very well and are attractive in design. They are called 'Kanga' because they have a pouch, like a kangaroo. The absorbent pad fits into this pouch. The pants have an elasticated waist and legs. The urine passes through the special knitted fabric of the pants into the pad in the pouch. This special fabric has a 'one-way only' effect with urine. Although the urine passes through it, you feel dry, as long as the pads are changed regularly. The pouch, on the outside of the pants, is made of woven fabric and is coated with plastic on the inside to make it waterproof. The pads are easy to place in position and remove. What is more, unlike some other pads, these do not need any fiddly things like press-studs or special fasteners. Leakage of urine and skin rashes are unlikely with these pads, provided you get a good fit. The pants should hug the body like a swimming costume. They are machine washable.

Pants to Avoid
Avoid ordinary plastic pants or giant-sized baby plastic pants. These are hard, uncomfortable to wear, and can be humiliating as they can make you feel like a baby. Because plastic prevents evaporation, they can cause perspiration, odour and skin rashes. If they fit badly, they can leak down the leg, or puddles can form in the gusset.

Recommended Pads
Kanga Pants should be worn with *Kanga Pads*, as they are specially designed for each other. Both are available direct from:

Kanga Hospital Products Ltd.
PO Box 39
Bentinck Street
BOLTON\BL1 4EX
(Tel: 0204-46226)

or:

Home Nursing Supplies Ltd.
Headquarters Road
West Wilts Trading Estate
WESTBURY Wiltshire
(Tel: 0373-822313)

Ordinary sanitary towels, designed for menstruation, may be adequate for slight dribbling of urine. Some are now designed to be highly absorbent, are slim, and stay dry on the side which touches the skin. A pad which is more absorbent than a sanitary towel, but looks like one, is the *Gelulose Pad*. This contains a substance which 'gels' when wet. It also contains a deodorant. It will absorb about three times as much fluid as an average pad of a similar size. Supplied by:

Gelulose Incontinence Products
91a King Street
SOUTHPORT
Merseyside PRQ 1LQ
(Tel: 0704 34518)

Disposable babies' nappies, the lightweight absorbent type, also work well and are not too bulky or obtrusive under clothes.

Various pads and pants suitable for moderate urine leakage are made by Molnlycke Ltd. A leaflet is available from:

Molnlycke Ltd.
Hospital Products Division
Station Approach
HARPENDEN
Hertfordshire AL5 4SR
(Tel: 05827 68111)

Pad to Avoid
Inco Roll – this is a big wodge of material on a roll. It disintegrates easily.

Note. No pads with pants will contain great gushes of urine. A catheter may be necessary if the flow of urine is always greater than can be contained by pads.

Aids for Men

Special incontinence sheaths have been designed for men, known as 'uridoms'. They look similar to contraceptive condoms. They fit snugly round the penis and are connected at the other end to a tube which leads to a plastic bag, which is strapped round the leg. The bag is emptied every so often. Men who are unable to fit an incontinence sheath have the same options of pads and pants as women. Some pants are designed like 'Y Fronts'. *Kanga Pants* make a particular style for men.

Incontinence sheaths are available from:

Seton Ltd.
Tubiton House
OLDHAM OL1 3HS

Men also have the advantage of being able to use urinals and other receptacles when a toilet is not at hand. (Receptacles for women do not work so well. One, called the

Feminal, handbag size personal urinal, has unfortunately not
done well in the St George's Hospital tests, as it is easy to miss
the receptacle opening unless it is placed accurately and with
a steady hand, with obvious results.)

Further Information about Aids for Incontinence

A very full and detailed list of commodes and chemical closets,
toilet aids, bath aids, receptacles, urinals, catheters, bags,
uridoms, pants and pads, bedpans, mattress protection, and
odour control, is given in a leaflet called *Notes on Incontinence*
published by:

> Disabled Living Foundation
> 346 Kensington High Street
> LONDON W14
> (Tel: 01-602 2491)

This is illustrated, and gives names and addresses of all
stockists.

The Disabled Living Foundation also has an Incontinence
Advisory Service, where you can ring or call in for advice.

Another good information leaflet is called *Incontinence* and is
published by:

> The Greater London Association for
>   the Disabled (GLAD)
> 1 Thorpe Close
> LONDON W10
> (Tel: 01-960 5799)

Action for Research into Multiple Sclerosis (ARMS) is
funding the research at St George's Hospital done by Morag
MacDougall. Her findings are available in a report called
Incontinence published by the ARMS Education Service and
available from:

> ARMS
> 71 Gray's Inn Road
> LONDON WC1

18 MENTAL OUTLOOK

Many people with M.S. find that the emotional and psychological problems that go with having the disease are a worse handicap than the disease itself, and more difficult to handle than physical defects.

Depression
Depression is a much more common reaction to a diagnosis of M.S. than euphoria, which has been said to go with having M.S.

Depression is most likely to happen soon after diagnosis when the full implications of the disease hit you. If you have seen people in advanced stages of the disease, or you have read medical text books about M.S., you may feel the worst is going to happen to you and so become awash with gloom and despair.

Many doctors tell their newly-diagnosed M.S. patients to 'go away and forget about it'. This kind of advice always makes me angry, but in a way you can see what they are getting at. They mean that you should not dwell on the worst possibilities or regard yourself as a cripple when you are not. The people with M.S. who have managed to acknowledge that they have the disease, yet carry on with as normal a life as possible, seem to suffer less from depression.

It is not easy to counteract depression, but one Australian woman I know of succeeded in overcoming it with a simple five-point plan.

—— Get plenty of sleep. Never get over-tired. (Notice how much more depressed you feel when you are tired.)
—— Eat often and plenty. Never let yourself get weak with hunger.
—— Exercise at least once a day.
—— Always have something to look forward to.
—— Be sociable. Take an interest in other people.

Add to that:

—— Think positively.
—— Take care to look good.
—— Stick to as ordered a routine as you can. Keep on top of things.
—— Keep your mind active and interested.
—— Do something that gives you a sense of achievement, for example, a creative hobby; helping other people in the community.
—— Live in the present and get the most out of each experience as it is actually happening. Do not dwell on the past or be fearful about the future.

Why Feeling Good is so Important

Recent research has shown that a family of chemicals called endorphins is produced in the brain when you are happy. Normal levels of endorphins are important to a feeling of well-being.

These endorphins are also thought to be associated with the release of certain hormones, like cortisol, which are involved in cell growth and the proper biological functioning of the body. It is thought that endorphins and the subsequent release of hormones like cortisol are low in people who have M.S. No one knows why. If the endorphins level in your brain is low, you are bound to feel depressed. Further, if you are feeling low, all the things that the endorphins trigger off in the body will be low too.

On the other hand, if the endorphins level in your brain is

high, like when you are in love and feel on top of the world, everything connected with it goes up too.

So, try and do things that give your mood a boost. Remember that feeling down in the dumps is going to hinder your health, never help it.

Your Attitude Towards Yourself

When you are told you have M.S., it is very difficult to go on thinking about yourself in quite the same way ever again. It is common that even in mild cases, where disability does not even show, the person feels 'disabled'. They feel they have stepped down from the status of the able-bodied.

It is easy to feel damaged, a psychological as well as a physical cripple; a second-rate person. Yet, this negative attitude is probably the most disabling thing of all. It is vital to fight it off.

I know some people with M.S. who are quite severely disabled; who walk with sticks or crutches and are occasionally in a wheelchair. Yet because they are always interested in other people, always smiling and with a joke up their sleeves, and have such appealing and attractive personalities, they are always the centre of attention and much in demand socially.

The most off-putting thing to other people is not that you walk with a limp, or that your hand shakes, but that you look downcast, grim-faced, embittered, or ready to bite anyone's head off if they speak to you.

To be a 'whole person' is hard at the best of times, but unless you accept yourself – which means a continual readjustment as the disease progresses – you cannot expect other people to accept you.

Self-esteem is your most vital asset. Somehow, people always think of you the same way you think of yourself. If you lack self-respect, you will not win respect from other people. If you are filled with self-loathing, you can be sure of a few enemies. If you have no love for yourself, no one else will be able to love you either. This is perhaps the hardest fact of life.

Some remarkable people who have been struck with M.S. have taken it as a blessing in disguise. They find it gives them the opportunity to find the true essence of life; to strip life of all its superficialities and banalities, and experience the true joy of living. They are the people who notice each petal on a flower and marvel at its beauty. Sometimes these people are religious, and find a solace in their particular God, but it is not essential to believe in God to feel this way. To enjoy the everyday beauty of life, you have to live in the present.

Balance

You may have lost your balance physically, but try to regain your balance psychologically. Maybe you are all work and no play. Maybe you have dormant talents which would develop the creative side of your personality if you awakened them.

If you make an effort to develop the sides of your personality you know are getting rusty, or just dormant, it will help increase your self-esteem. Many people are over-balanced towards the materialistic side of life, to the detriment of the spiritual side, but are happier once they redress this imbalance.

Grief

A sense of loss is very common after you have been told you have M.S. It is as if a part of you has died, and you naturally mourn and grieve for it. The period of bereavement for your old self will take time. A new you will emerge, but it will not be exactly the same person as you were before. You may have to go through an agonizing period spanning the emotions of shock, bewilderment, terror, anger and rage before a calmer you emerges.

Body Image

Everybody who has M.S. can remember what they were like before they had it. Everyone with M.S. was at one time fit and healthy, able to run around, climb mountains, play sports, and sprint to catch a bus. When all those things become impossible, your body image changes, sometimes dramatically.

People with M.S. may come to see themselves as no longer useful or attractive to others. They must also learn to live with what is still the stigma of M.S. A poor self-image can cause them to fear rejection by their partner, or prospective partners, and those kinds of fears have a nasty way of being self-fulfilling prophesies.

It is important to try and keep hold of a positive body image. There is no reason why you cannot still take good care of your appearance and dress stylishly, even on a low budget. Many women I know with M.S. are beautiful and elegant, even though they may be in a wheelchair or walking with the aid of sticks.

Coming to Terms with M.S.

This is extraordinarily difficult, as M.S. keeps on changing. You may come to terms with one set of disabilities, when another disability comes along, and the whole process of 'coming to terms' has to start again. Readjustment is a never-ending process, an ever-changing challenge.

If you can be realistic about your situation, your bitterness and disappointment will be less. Life is unpredictable anyway; M.S. just makes it more so.

'Invisible' Symptoms

These symptoms include fatigue; weak, blurred or double vision; and difficulties with bladder control.

With symptoms like these, it is relatively easy to hide from the rest of the world the fact that you have got M.S., and you may try and deceive yourself too, with the result that you end up in a state of conflict about your own indentity. It could also add to your stress and anxiety, which could well make things worse. It is probably better not to deny something that is evidently true.

19 RELATIONSHIPS AND SEX

If you already have an intimate and loving relationship with your partner, there is no reason why M.S. should threaten the relationship; indeed, it could well bring you closer together.

On the other hand, a chronic and potentially disabling illness like M.S. can throw a severe strain on a relationship which lacks deep intimacy and communication. If the person with M.S. finds it difficult to talk freely and difficult to accept help, or is very demanding; or if the partner is unable to offer help, then a marriage could be in dire straits.

When either a husband or wife gets M.S., it is difficult to carry on with family life as if nothing has happened. On the other hand, the person with M.S. does not want to be labelled an invalid, and give up the role of wife, mother, husband, father, or breadwinner.

Even though your body image may have changed, you are still you. You are still able to give and receive love, to laugh, cry, share emotions, and be needed by your family, friends and colleagues. You will feel more of a sense of worth if you keep reminding yourself that you are needed, loved and lovable.

If you go around being a misery and a grump, you will find

it difficult to like yourself, and you can hardly expect others to either. A frown puts people off, but a smile attracts.

You can control your moods if you decide to. It is better to try and take a light-hearted approach to M.S. problems than a heavy-handed, gloomy one. Certainly, they are no joke, but the people I know with M.S. who can manage to make a joke out of their difficulties tend to get on much better in life than those who do not. They are the kind of people who might chuckle 'Oh! There I go, peeing again' when they are incontinent, rather than being shamefully embarrassed about it.

Relationship Problems
It is easy to turn M.S. into the scapegoat for all marital and sexual problems, when it is the basic relationship itself that is at fault.

Even so, M.S. is going to dramatically affect any relationship. Feelings that neither of you may have had to confront before are likely to hit you with a terrible impact: feelings of fear, frustration, rage, perhaps hostility and guilt.

Each couple must work out for themselves the issues of dependence and independence – to what extent the one with M.S. can make demands on the other, and to what extent the one without M.S. should give help to the other. Some sufferers will fall into the 'sick' role, and use it to manipulate their partners or other relatives, but this will only make them feel guilt and hostility.

These issues are very hard to deal with, but they must be confronted and talked through. It may be necessary to get help from a professional therapist or counsellor.

Children
Children can be very bewildered and shocked by a parent who gets M.S. They may have had a mum who used to run round the park with them, or a dad who played football, but cannot any longer.

What and when you tell them depends on their age, but the key is to be honest. Try not to tell a four-year-old more than he can understand. Instinctively, children are aware that something is wrong and that you are worried. You need to be aware of this and understand that their behaviour can sometimes be disturbed. They need comfort and reassurance.

Your children may have to alter their views about what mothers and fathers are supposed to be like, and this adjustment will take time.

Older children may appear outwardly calm or even indifferent when they are told you have M.S., yet inwardly they could be acutely anxious about it. The way to deal with this is to talk to them, giving them a little information at a time rather than one long talk. Treat them as adults, and let them play a responsible part in family life.

Telling Other People

What you tell other people may depend on the extent of your disability. You might feel comfortable telling some people, but not others.

It may surprise you how helpful some of the people you tell turn out to be. Be as matter-of-fact as possible. Try not to cast yourself in the great 'tragic' role, or the medical bore.

On the other hand, there may be some people with whom it is wise to be reticent. It requires courage to come out into the open with a disease that unfortunately still carries a social stigma. The danger with telling some people is that you get labelled as 'the person with M.S.', and it is quite a challenge to surpass this limiting label.

Who Do You Turn to for Help?

A husband, wife or parent is probably not the best person to turn to. After all, they are suffering too, with similar feelings of loss, grief, and fear. Cry together – but not on their shoulder. It does not always follow that the 'unaffected' partner is the strong one. So it is better to turn to someone outside the immediate situation.

It is important that you do pour your heart out to somebody. The worst thing you can do is bottle it up inside yourself – that would only add to your anxiety.

So, who can you turn to?

ARMS Telephone Counselling Service

England and Wales: 01-568 2255
Scotland: 041-637 2262

Action for Research into Multiple Sclerosis is a self-help pressure group and charity where all the members have M.S., or have a close relative with M.S. They run a very good twenty-four-hour telephone counselling service, manned by trained counsellors who either have M.S. themselves or are closely related to someone who has. They are there to listen to any problems concerning M.S., at any time of the day or night, any day of the year, from M.S. sufferers, their family, or friends. The counsellors help callers cope with their distress, fears and anger and try and help them find hope for the future.

Social Workers
If you do not have a social worker already, contact the Social Services Department of your local council and they will organize it. A social worker should be able to help you with practical advice, and can advise on aids, adaptations to your home, home helps etc. Your local council should also be able to send a health visitor when you need one.

Multiple Sclerosis Society Welfare Officer
If you are a member of the M.S. Society of Great Britain and Northern Ireland, they have a welfare officer who could help you with practical problems. Ask your branch secretary, or write to their head office.

286 Munster Road
LONDON SW6 6AP
(Tel: 01-381 4022/3/4/5)

Psychotherapists
If you find yourself overwhelmed by depression as a result of having M.S., your doctor should be able to refer you to a good psychotherapist. In some cases it is possible, though difficult, to get psychotherapy free on the National Health Service (in the U.K.). Even though psychotherapy is very time-consuming, and can go on for years, it is worth considering if your personal relationship with your partner or any other problem is giving you distress and you are unable to sort it all out on your own.

Sexual Problems in Men and Women
There is no reason why M.S. should stop or limit your sexual relationship with your partner, or prevent you being a person with sexual desires and needs.

It is true that M.S. can cause specific sexual problems, but with love, information, communication, an open attitude, patience, and perhaps with the help of new positions or sexual aids, these can be overcome.

It is very important if you are the one with M.S. that your partner goes on seeing you as a sexually attractive person, and you must do everything to keep yourself that way.

If you think you are unattractive, or doubt your ability to attract or keep a partner, it will have a devastating effect on your self-image and self-esteem. So it is vital to accept and love yourself, so others can feel that way about you too.

Your definition of sexuality may have to be broadened beyond the ability or inability just to have sexual intercourse.

To overcome sex problems you have to communicate openly and honestly with your partner. If you do not share your feelings, your partner may not be aware of your needs. Love and patience on the part of both partners seldom fails to solve problems.

The worst thing you can do is avoid sexual contact. Some couples have a tendency to do this because they are afraid that sex will worsen the condition of the one with M.S. On the other hand, they may avoid sex because they do not want it to end in disappointment or frustration, if this has been the out-come of previous encounters.

The danger is that if you become too watchful or worried about what might go wrong, this 'spectatoring' in itself becomes a problem. Performance anxieties always interfere with relaxation and enjoyment, and can inhibit an erection in men and orgasm in women.

Fatigue

This is a major problem for both men and women with M.S. However, it is possible to counteract fatigue being a sex problem if you plan your sex life beforehand, even though this does mean that sex will not be spontaneous.

Choose a time of day for sex when your energy is at its highest. It is silly to have sex late at night when you have no energy left. If you make love during the day, rest beforehand. If necessary, get your neighbours to take the children. Avoid interruptions. Try and create a relaxing and erotic atmosphere, it will help make it a more satisfying sexual encounter.

Problems in Men

In men, neurological damage can give rise to partial or complete impotence, though emotional factors may be responsible for lack of erection, on some occasions. Like any other M.S. symptoms, potency can go away and then come back again.

Men may experience anything from minor difficulties in getting and keeping an erection, to disturbances of sensation and ejaculation, to total failure to get an erection.

Ejaculation may be affected because it is also a reflex controlled by the bundle of nerves in the lower spinal cord. Men who have difficulty getting or keeping an erect penis may be less likely to ejaculate.

Problems in Women

Women with M.S. *may* suffer loss of orgasm, diminished libido or spasticity. They may also have problems with reduced lubrication, anxiety about bladder control, and fatigue. On the other hand, many women with quite severe disability do not experience any of these things, and enjoy normal, satisfying sex.

Intercourse may be more difficult because of spasms of the thighs, and reduced vaginal lubrication. An artificial lubricant, like *KY Jelly*, usually solves this.

Many women with M.S. continue to have a normal orgasm reflex. Others, depending on the extent of their neurological damage, may not experience genital orgasm. But it is thought possible for women who do not have a physiological orgasm to nevertheless reach a psychological climax – a sort of 'phantom' orgasm, following the partner's excitement and orgasm and sharing a common tension release.

Overcoming Sexual Problems

Even though sexual intercourse may be hard to achieve, many people find the emotional and psychological pleasure of it vital to a relationship, and it is worth striving to overcome specific difficulties for this reason.

If a man has erection difficulties, intercourse can be achieved by the woman sitting astride her partner and placing his flaccid penis inside her vagina. If she voluntarily contracts her vaginal muscles around his penis, she can hopefully bring about a partial erection.

It may be necessary to try new and different positions to accommodate the partner's specific problems. It should be possible to find a position which is comfortable, and gives pleasure and satisfaction to both partners.

Catheters can be taped against the body so that they are out of the way. A man can wear a condom for hygiene.

If intercourse is too difficult, there are other sexual possibilities to maintain intimacy with your partner. Anything that gives mutual pleasure should be considered right and good, despite some people's attitudes that they might be 'perverted'. These would include oral sex, masturbation, and of course massaging, cuddling, fondling or any other means of touching and mutual caressing. In a healthy sexual relationship, these would be all additions to sexual intercourse, and not alternatives.

Sexual aids can give pleasure and satisfaction in lovemaking, so you should not treat them with suspicion just because they are manufactured and not 'natural'. Anything that does not actually cause pain in sex, and which gives pleasure to both partners should be welcomed rather than shunned. After all, no one minds wearing glasses if their eyesight is poor; the same attitude should apply to sexual aids.

If you are embarrassed by the prospect of going into a sex shop, such items can be obtained by mail order. Write to SPOD (see below) for a list of suppliers of sex aids.

Where to Go for Help with Sexual Problems

There is an organization specifically set up to help disabled people with their sex problems. It is called SPOD (Sexual and Relationship Problems of the Disabled), and the address is:

SPOD
25 Mortimer Street
LONDON W1N 8AB
(Tel: 01-637 5400)

SPOD publishes a series of very good and helpful advisory leaflets. For example:

—— *Physically Handicapped People and Sex.*
—— *Physical Handicap and Sexual Intercourse: Positions for Sex.*
—— *Physical Handicap and Sexual Intercourse: Methods and Techniques.*

—— *Aids to Sex for the Physically Handicapped.*
—— *Sex for the Severely Disabled.*
—— *Your Disabled Partner and Sex.*

There is also a good booklet published by the Multiple Sclerosis Society of Canada called *Sexuality and Multiple Sclerosis* which you can get direct from SPOD. SPOD also provides an advisory and counselling service for disabled people in sexual difficulty. They also have a list of suppliers of sex aids.

Psychosexual Counselling
This is now widely available at many family planning clinics. If you are too shy to ask your doctor where to go, contact any Family Planning Association branch, or the National Marriage Guidance Council, both of whom do sex counselling. This type of counselling is for sex problems which are fundamentally psychological. This may be the case even where physical disease is involved.

FURTHER READING

General

A Manual on Multiple Sclerosis by Helmut J. Bauer (International Federation of Multiple Sclerosis Societies). Available from: ARMS, 71 Gray's Inn Road, London WC1X 8TR.

'Multiple Sclerosis' in *British Medical Bulletin*. Available from: Medical Department, The British Council, 65 Davis Street, London W1Y 2AA.

Multiple Sclerosis: A Reappraisal by D. McAlpine, C. Lumsden and D. Acheson (Churchill Livingstone).

Multiple Sclerosis Research by Medical Research Council. Available from: H.M. Stationery Offices. London: 49 High Holborn, WC1V 6HB.

Multiple Sclerosis: The Facts by W.B. Matthews (Oxford University Press, 1980).

Multiple Sclerosis. (Part of a self-help guide series.) Available from: Lunesdale Publishing Group Limited, Lunesdale House, Hornby, Lancaster, Lancs.

Management of M.S.

A Guide to the Management of Multiple Sclerosis: Naudicelle, Dietary, Exercise by Joe Osborne. Available from: Joe Osborne, 24 Beech Grove, Newhall, Burton-on-Trent, Staffs.

Living with Multiple Sclerosis by Dr Elizabeth Forsythe (Faber, 1979).

Exercise

Multiple Sclerosis: Control of the Disease by W. Ritchie-Russell (Pergamon Press, 1976).

Multiple Sclerosis: Simple Exercises by Gill Robinson. Available from: ARMS or the M.S. Society (see *Useful Addresses*).

The Articulate Body by Sidi Hessel (New English Library, 1979).

Diet

The Low-Fat Gourmet: A Doctor's Cookbook for Heart Diseases and M.S. by Dr Elizabeth Forsythe (Pelham Books).

The Multiple Sclerosis Diet Book by Professor Roy Swank. Available from: ARMS (see *Useful Addresses*).

Good Food, Gluten-Free by Hilda Cherry Hill. Available from: Henry Doubleday Research Association, Bocking, Braintree, Essex.

Rita Greer's Extraordinary Kitchen Notebook

Fruit and Vegetables in Particular

The First Clinical Ecology Cookbook

All by Rita Greer and available from: Roberts Publications, 225 Putney Bridge Road, London SW15 2PY.

Help Fight M.S.: Dietary Therapy with Polyunsaturated Fatty Acids by Dr Paul Evers. Available from: Klinik Dr Evers, 5768 Sundern-Langsheid, West Germany.

Manual of Nutrition by Ministry of Agriculture, Fisheries and Food. Available from: H.M. Stationery Offices.

Dietary Fats and Oils in Human Nutrition by Food and Agricultural Organization. Available from: H.M. Stationery Offices.

What We Eat Today by Michael and Sheilagh Crawford (Spearman, 1968).

Minerals and Your Health by Len Mervyn (Allen & Unwin, 1980).

Minerals: What They Are and Why We Need Them by Miriam Polunin (Thorsons, 1979).

Sex
Sexuality and Multiple Sclerosis by Michael Barrett Ph.D. Available from: Multiple Sclerosis Society of Canada or SPOD (see *Useful Addresses*).

Entitled to Love by Wendy Greengross (Malaby Press in association with the National Fund for Research into Crippling Diseases). Available from: Malaby Press Limited, Aldine House, 26 Albemarle Street, London W1.

Newsletters, Information and Booklets
ARMS Education Service booklets:

Pain in M.S. by Dr Keith Budd.

A View on Diet by Rita Greer.

Fatigue by Professor D. Edholm and Dr A. Burnfield.

M.S.: A World Review by Professor H.J. Bauer.

Nutrition in M.S. by Professor Roy Swank.

Also *ARMS Link* newsletter, sent free to ARMS members. Full of new information and helpful hints. Available from: ARMS (see *Useful Addresses*).

M.S. Society News. A quarterly bulletin available free to members – newsy helpful and informative. Available from: M.S. Society of Great Britain and Northern Ireland (see *Useful Addresses*).

General Books for the Disabled

Coping with Disablement by Peggy Jay. Available from: Consumer's Association, 14 Buckingham Street, London WC2N 6DS.

Directory for the Disabled, compiled by Ann Darnborough and Derek Kinrade. (Published in association with the Multiple Sclerosis Society of G.B. and Northern Ireland by Woodhead-Faulkner Ltd., 8 Market Passage, Cambridge CB2 3PF.

Better Lives for Disabled Women by Jo Campling (Virago).

The Source Book for the Disabled, edited by Glorye Hale (Paddington Press).

Other Relevant Books

Let's Get Well by Adelle Davis (Allen & Unwin, 1974).

Let's Eat Right to Keep Fit by Adelle Davis (Allen & Unwin, 1974).

Not All in the Mind by Dr Richard Mackarness (Pan Books, 1976).

Reflexology by Anna Kaye and Don C. Matchan (Thorsons, 1979).

Reflexology Today: Healing Through Your Feet by Doreen Bayly. Available from: The Humane Education Centre, Avenue Lodge, Bounds Green Road, London N22 4EU.

Yoga and Health by Selvarajan Yesudian and Elisabeth Haich (Allen & Unwin, 1978).

USEFUL ADDRESSES

ARMS (Action for Research into Multiple Sclerosis)
71 Gray's Inn Road
LONDON WC1X 8TR

ARMS Research Unit
Central Middlesex Hospital
Acton Lane
Park Royal
LONDON NW10
(Tel: 01-961 4911 or 01-965 5733 ext. 627)

Advice on diet, exercise, counselling, plus library for ARMS
    members.

ARMS Telephone Counselling Service.
England and Wales:
    Tel: 01-568 2255
Scotland:
    Tel: 041-637 2262
Twenty-four hours a day, seven days a week, all year service.
For anyone suffering from M.S. or their family and friends.
Manned by trained counsellors who know about M.S. from
personal experience.

Multiple Sclerosis Society of Great Britain and Northern
Ireland
286 Munster Road
LONDON SW6 6AP
(Tel: 01-381 4022/3/4/5)

The Disabled Living Foundation
346 Kensington High Street
LONDON W14
(Tel: 01-602 2491)

Details about aids and equipment.

The Disability Alliance
1 Cambridge Terrace
LONDON NW1 4JL
(Tel: 01-935 4992)

Publishes, *Disability Rights Handbook.*

Burton and South Derbyshire Independent Pool for the
Sufferers of M.S.
24 Beech Grove
Newhall
BURTON-ON-TRENT
Staffordshire
(Tel: 0283 216638)

Sexual and Personal Relations of the Disabled (SPOD)
c/o Royal Association for Disability and Rehabilitation
(RADAR)
25 Mortimer Street
LONDON W1N 8AB
(Tel: 01-637 5400)

Bio Oil Research Ltd (for *Naudicelle*)
Royal Oak Building
High Street
CREWE
Cheshire CW2 7BL
(Tel: 0270-213094)

Efamol Ltd (for *Efamol G*)
40 Warton Road
LONDON E15 2JU
(Tel: 01-555 9042-7)

Action Against Allergy
43 The Downs
LONDON SW20 8HG
(Tel: 01-947 5082)

International Federation of Multiple Sclerosis Societies
Stubenring 6
A-1010 Vienna
AUSTRIA
(Tel: 528864)

Multiple Sclerosis Societies Around the World

Australia
National Multiple Sclerosis Society of Australia
127 Collins Street
MELBOURNE 3000
Victoria

Austria
Osterreichische MS Gesellschaft
Lazarettgasse 14
A-1090 WIEN

Belgium
Ligue Belge de la Sclerose en Plaques
A.S.B.L.
188 Avenue Plasky
BRUSSELS 1040

Canada
Multiple Sclerosis Society of Canada
Suite 700
130 Bloor Street West
TORONTO
Ontario M5S IN9.

Denmark
Landsforeningen til Bekjempelse af Dissemineret Sclerose
Rosenborggade 5
1130 COPENHAGEN K

Finland
Finlands M.S.-Foreningars Forbund
r.v. Venalhontie
21250 MASKU

France
Comité National de la Sclerose en Plaques
17 Boulevard Auguste-Blanque
F 75013
PARIS

Germany
Deutsch Multiple Sclerose Gesellschaft, E.V.
9 FRANKFURT-AM-MAIN
Auf der Kornerwiese 5

Ireland
The Multiple Sclerosis Society of Ireland
14 Merrion Square
DUBLIN 2.

Israel
Israel M.S. Society
10 Esther Hamlka Street
TEL AVIV

Italy
Associazione Italiana Sclerosi Multiple
Via della Magliana 279
00 146 ROMA

Netherlands
Nederland Multiple Sclerosis Stiching
Bezuidenhoutsweg 299
DEN HAAG

New Zealand
The National Multiple Sclerosis Society of New Zealand Inc.
Suite 501
Fifth Floor
D.I.C. Building
WELLINGTON

Norway
Multiple Sklerose-Forbundet i Norge
Jac
Aallsgate 26
OSLO 3.

South Africa
South African National Multiple Sclerosis Society
295 Villiers Road
Walmer
PORT ELIZABETH

Sweden
MS-Forbundet
David Bagares Gate 3
S-111 38 STOCKHOLM

Switzerland
Schweizerische Multiple Sclerose Ges.
Forchstrasse 55
8032 ZURICH

United States of America
National Multiple Sclerosis Society
205 East 42nd Street
NEW YORK 10017

INDEX

160   MULTIPLE SCLEROSIS